Whether you are still in the process of deciding on a therapy, about to begin treatment, or already on it, it is important to remember that many people before you have gone through chemo, that they did manage to cope, and that there are ways that have been developed to help you get through it, too. The same strength that stems from the will to live and enables people to make the tough decision to undergo chemo continues to stand them in good stead during the actual treatment. So do a positive attitude, a good doctor-patient relationship, and a realistic picture of what to expect in the way of results and side effects.

We all learn to cope because we have to—the alternative is much worse. We choose chemotherapy because no matter what the price we pay—in time, money, side effects, and emotional energy—the benefits are greater than without it. Ultimately it is something within ourselves that allows us to make the extra effort to tough it out.

Coping
With
Chemotherapy

Nancy Bruning

BALLANTINE BOOKS • NEW YORK

Library of Congress Catalog Card Number: 84-9612

ISBN 0-345-33090-0

This edition published by arrangement with Doubleday and Company, Inc.

Manufactured in the United States of America

First Ballantine Books Edition: April 1986

*I would like to dedicate this book to my husband,
my oncologist, my mother, and my friends—
all of whom, in their own ways,
helped me find the strength to cope with chemotherapy.
And to you, the chemotherapy patient,
who helped me find the strength to write it.*

●●●●●● ACKNOWLEDGMENTS

There are so many people who believed in this book and helped me in so many ways that I scarcely know where to begin to offer my appreciation.

Perhaps at the beginning, to my editor, Fran McCullough, and my agent, Susan Protter, whose encouragement and guidance were instrumental in its inception and indispensable to its completion. Also to my husband, Michael Gross, and to my good friend Kathleen O'Reilly, who read the manuscript, understood the magnitude of the task, and offered valuable support and suggestions when I needed them most.

To the cancer patients who shared with me their experiences with chemotherapy in the hope that others might benefit from them.

My thanks—and admiration—to the oncologists and other cancer care professionals at various cancer centers who graciously took time from their busy schedules to answer my questions and read parts of the manuscript.

From Memorial Sloan-Kettering Cancer Center: Grace Christ, director of the Department of Social Work; Dr. Thomas Fahey, deputy chief medical officer of the Outpatient Department; Dr. Richard Gralla, associate attending physician; Dr. Thomas Hakes, assistant attending physician; Patricia Henry, oncology nurse; Linda James, planning analyst in the Department of

Strategic Planning; Matthew Loscalzo, social worker; Sister Rosemary Moynihan, social work supervisor; and Donna Park, assistant director of nursing, Ambulatory Care.

From the Denver Presbyterian Medical Center: Pam Felling, staff physical therapist; M.L. Frohling, biofeedback technician; Lisa Logan, clinical dietician; and Regina Schmidt, oncology nurse/team coordinator.

From St. Vincent's Hospital and Medical Center: Dr. Judith Bukberg, chief of Consultation-Liaison Psychiatry; and Dr. William Grace, chief of oncology.

Special thanks to New York oncologist Dr. Ward F. Cunningham-Rundles, Los Angeles oncologist Dr. Michael Van Scoy-Mosher, and Dr. Ronald Bash of Albert Einstein Hospital—all extraordinary oncologists and remarkable human beings.

I would also like to thank the following: Barbara Blumberg, Linda Anderson, and Betty MacVicar from the National Cancer Institute; Dr. Michael Schachter of the Mountainview Medical Associates; Dr. Philip Schulman, oncologist at North Shore University Hospital; Katherine Crosson, director of Patient Education at M.D. Anderson University of Texas Cancer Center; Patricia Fobaire, radiation social worker at Stanford University Medical Center; Dr. James A. Niedhart, chairman of the Department of Medical Oncology at M.D. Anderson Hospital and Tumor Institute, the University of Texas System Cancer Center; Dr. Maryl Winningham, exercise physiologist at the Ohio State University Center for Nursing Research; Dr. Charles Vogel, director of the Comprehensive Cancer Center for the State of Florida; Lari Wenzel, former director of the Cancer Information Service and rehabilitation coordinator for the Comprehensive Cancer Center for the State of Florida; Sylvia Weissman, associate director of Social Services at Cancer Care, Inc.; Shari Lieberman, New York dietician and nutritionist; Lin Perkin, Denver exercise physiologist; Mr. Nicholas, wig stylist for the Kenneth Beauty Salon in New York; Joseph Rodriguez, general manager of the Vidal Sassoon Salon in New York; and Edith Imre, proprietor of Edith Imre Hair Fashions, Inc.

●●●●● CONTENTS

In 1980, at the age of thirty-one, I discovered I had breast cancer. A biopsy had revealed that the lump that had grown alarmingly large over the last few months was not a cyst—it was a malignancy. In order to save my life—so my surgeon said—I had to have the standard surgical procedure, a modified radical mastectomy, the very next day. Although this removed all the visible tumor, unfortunately some lymph nodes were involved and this meant that the cancer might have spread to other parts of my body. The only way to kill these stray cancer cells was with chemotherapy, which I was advised to have "just in case."

Without a doubt, I found the idea of chemotherapy more frightening than the surgery I had just been through. The fact was, in spite of major, mutilating, and supposedly life-saving surgery, my surgeon might not have "gotten it all." It wasn't over yet: Cancer might still be somewhere in my body, and I was now being offered a treatment about which I knew very little and what little I did know was all bad. I had allowed my surgeon to lop off my breast without investigating my options, and it hadn't worked. I felt betrayed and, mistrustful of medical advice, was not about to be rushed into something else I didn't know a lot about.

So I went to a chemotherapist other than the one recommended by my surgeon. Through sheer luck—referral from a friend of a friend who also had cancer—I found a capable, compassionate cancer specialist whom I liked, respected, and trusted immediately. (And during the course of treatment I grew to like, respect, and trust him even more.) He explained the statistics: Without chemotherapy my chances of remaining disease-free for ten years would be about 15 percent; according to the latest scientific study, published in 1979, the best standard chemotherapy increased my chances to about 70 percent—at least for the next eight years. He described the course of therapy—the scheduling of the drugs and their likely side effects —and then assured me he would do everything he knew, nutritionally and otherwise, to help minimize the side effects. Clearly, 70 percent was better than 15 percent; a quick assessment of the unorthodox therapies revealed no comparative figures, which made those therapies more frightening than chemo. Under the circumstances, I agreed to the plan. I wanted to live, and chemo seemed the best chance there was.

Were I in a position to have to do it all over again, I would. Looking back, chemotherapy was not as bad as I had thought it would be. I continued to work and enjoy most of my usual activities, even though I didn't feel exactly wonderful. I had a relatively hopeful prognosis, I got low-dose chemo under the care of a good physician, and I was surrounded by people who cared. Everyone thought I coped amazingly well, and I suppose I did. But I know I would have coped even better if I had done some things a little differently.

I realize now what I didn't then, while I was busy grappling with the real possibility of my own death: that I should have been better informed about my disease and its treatment; that I should have been better prepared to deal with some of the side effects, especially the complete hair loss; that I needed even more emotional support than my doctor, family, and friends could give; and that I did not have to suffer alone in my feelings of depression, anxiety, doubt, fear, anger, confusion, sadness, ignorance, and isolation.

I know too that a book about chemotherapy would have been a great help and comfort to me. In the two years that passed after I completed my own chemo, several excellent books on cancer and its treatment were published, but there was still nothing for the general audience that focused solely on chemotherapy and how to get through it. And so the idea and the conviction to write a book on coping with chemotherapy came about, a book based in part on the methods that I found successful, and in part on the experiences of others.

Throughout my research—as I absorbed (or tried to absorb) the medical literature and spoke with over fifty cancer specialists, social workers, nurses, and cancer patients all over the country—I learned that chemotherapy is a highly individual matter. There are hundreds of different chemotherapy treatments; and people's diseases, personalities, life circumstances, prognoses, levels of tolerance, and reactions to the drugs can and do vary. So do the will to live and the ability to fight.

Chemotherapy is clearly not for everyone, but anyone who is faced with its mixed blessings should be fully informed before making any decisions about it. No one should accept or refuse, or continue or stop, chemotherapy out of ignorance or fear. The cruel facts are that there are patients who might be helped by chemotherapy but who are not getting it; that there are those who might be better helped by it; and that there are some who are harmed rather than helped by chemotherapy and who shouldn't be getting it at all.

The chemotherapy experience can fall short of what it might be—how it can be used, how it can benefit, and the degree of comfort the patient maintains while undergoing it—because chemotherapy patients suddenly find themselves plunged into a maze without a map. Cancer care for most people is completely foreign territory—full of half-truths, myths, and misconceptions; of personal issues and dilemmas; of complicated new words and procedures; of hot and cold running hope and fear.

But chemotherapy is not what it used to be. If it is given wisely and well to informed patients, chemo can cure some people and extend the comfortable productive life-spans of many others.

Most cancer patients do learn to cope with their disease and their treatment in their own ways, using whatever works best for them. But the coping process can always be made easier, swifter, and better. There are many ways to make sure that you get the best chemo available and to help you get through it as easily as possible. There are ways and people to make your treatment less formidable, to help you, your family, and your friends meet your challenges from positions of strength rather than of weakness. As a chemotherapy patient you are in dire

need of *information* in order to be able to weigh your options
sensibly. You need *guidance* so you can help your cancer specialist help you. You need *practical suggestions* to make living
under chemotherapy more comfortable. Most of all you need
to be *reassured* that others have entered the special world of
chemotherapy, have come out the other end, and are managing
to adapt to the new life the experience has presented to them.
And this is what I hope this book will provide.

Ideally, *Coping with Chemotherapy* should be read from
beginning to end. But this is a less than ideal world and you're
probably not too interested in the history of chemotherapy if
your hair has just begun to fall out in handfuls. Take from this
book what you need, when you need it. Remember that chemotherapy is a young, fast-changing field, so this book is by no
means the final word on this treatment. Nor can it take the
place of a qualified physician or other health care professional.

Coping with Chemotherapy is a supplement to your doctor's
care and a resource for the many other aspects of cancer in
which you may be interested. The book necessarily concen-
trates on those aspects that are most directly related to the issue
at hand—chemotherapy. But where does cancer end and chemotherapy begin? Chemotherapy does not exist in a vacuum: A
chemo patient is after all a cancer patient. I have touched briefly
upon many areas that concern all cancer patients in the hope
that this will pique further interest and self-education in this
endlessly fascinating subject that will on some level be of
concern for the rest of our lives. Volumes have been written
about areas I have kept brief, for example, about other forms
of therapy and psychosocial concerns. I have also stayed away
from childhood cancer, because that is a whole other world
that could not have been treated adequately here. Many sources
of information about these and related subjects are listed in the
Appendix, to which you might want to refer.

Anyone facing chemotherapy surely has a big job ahead.
The physical and psychological changes and challenges in your
life begin at the time of diagnosis; they may come to a peak
sometime during the treatment; and they can continue for long
afterward. It is not an easy road you travel, and it may often
be a lonely one. *Coping with Chemotherapy* was written for
you to turn to again and again, whenever you need information,
inspiration, or simply a hand to hold. I hope you will be able
to draw strength, comfort, courage, assurance, and wisdom
from these pages and the people who have contributed of them-

selves in order to help others who are going through a similar difficult time. But no matter how much help you have, it is still up to you and your own strength and determination to make it as you pick your own way along the path to coping with chemotherapy.

Should You Have
Chemotherapy?

Coping with chemotherapy begins with the decision to undergo it. This decision is not an easy one, but then important decisions rarely are. Though you may rely on others for information and advice, ultimately the choice is up to you.

However, whether you are on the threshold of chemotherapy or already well into it, the choice to begin and/or the choice to continue can be made much more easily and more responsibly.

Many patients and cancer care professionals find, for instance, that learning something about cancer is the first step in a sound decision-making process. An understanding of what chemotherapy is, how it works, and its advantages and shortcomings is also essential, as are a realistic picture of its goals, your prognosis, your alternatives, and how chemotherapy fits in with and compares to other forms of treatment. You also need to find a competent, caring cancer specialist (oncologist) who will be responsive to your needs and who will give you the most effective treatment with the least possible side effects. Access to the many methods used to support chemotherapy patients is also paramount.

Admittedly, some of these factors carry more weight than others, depending upon the individual. But all contribute to your making informed, intelligent choices throughout your therapy, to a basic conviction that you are doing the right thing, and to your having a feeling of control over your life. These are all fundamental to accepting treatment and learning to live with it.

CHAPTER 1

Understanding Cancer

No one can expect to become a cancer specialist overnight, but acquiring a basic understanding of your disease is worth the effort and is a necessary preliminary to understanding all cancer therapies. Dr. Richard Gralla, an oncologist who specializes in lung cancer at Memorial Sloan-Kettering in New York City, says:

"In a society where astrology is more known than astronomy, where every other corner has a tarot card reader, people don't want to be faced with the difficult technological problems. Yet they want to understand why you can't cure cancer. People try to understand cancer without understanding very much about biology in general. I think people do not understand their disease because they don't understand a little of the basic science that goes into it. And yet you hear people complain that when your doctor tells you something, you have no choice; you have to listen to him. What choice do you have if you don't know very much about these things in general? The degree of knowledge necessary is that which is taught on a junior high school or perhaps ninth or tenth grade level."

CELL BIOLOGY

Your body is made up of many different types of tissue—
skin, muscle, bone, blood, glands, and other organs. The tissues in turn are made up of tiny specialized cells that perform
specific functions. Within each cell is a *nucleus* that contains
chromosomes: There are twenty-three sets of "regular chromosomes" and one set of "sex chromosomes." Each chromosome can contain up to several thousand genes. The genes in
turn are made up of *deoxyribonucleic acid* (DNA), which takes
the form of two spiraling strands. The DNA can be likened to
a foreman who controls the cell's activities; it is the DNA that
ultimately makes up the genetic program of each cell.

One of the activities that the DNA oversees is that of reproduction. Cells reproduce themselves in order to replace those
that have become damaged or have died, or if more cells are
needed for some special reason. Some cells, like those making
up the blood, are replaced more often than others. For example,
the white blood cells are replaced completely every six hours,
a rate of production that is stepped up during infection, when
a greater than normal quantity of them is needed.

Cells reproduce by division—one cell splits in half to produce a "daughter" cell. There is a time in every cell's life when
it reproduces; there is a time when it is "fertile" and a time
when it is not. Cells go through four phases during each of
their reproductive cycles in which the DNA makes an exact
copy of itself to pass on to the nucleus of the next generation.
Some types of cells reproduce within hours; others may take
days, weeks, months, or years. After division, the cell begins
the next four-phase reproductive cycle, perhaps after first passing through a resting phase.

Normal human cells are obedient and altruistic. They "know"
when they should reproduce and when they should not. They
stay where they belong. They perform whatever functions they
are programmed to perform. Whatever their functions and rates
of growth, they are for the good of the entire body. (Cells also
respond to other stimuli such as the commands given by the
hormones produced in our endocrine glands.)

Cancer cells, however, do not obey the various commands
of the body. Unlike normal cells, whose motto might be One

for All and All for One, cancer cells behave as if it's Every Man for Himself. They reproduce wildly, more often than the normal cells that surround them. They are usually unable to perform any useful function for the good of the entire body. On the contrary, they are *malignant*, meaning they invade and injure vital organs of the body, thus interfering with those organs' ability to perform needed functions. In advanced stages of cancer, these cells spread and grow in other parts of the body to wreak havoc there too.

Though they arise from normal cells, cancer cells usually don't look like the other cells in the tissue of origin. They may be oddly misshapen, have a strange membrane or nucleus, or contain the wrong number of chromosomes.

CAUSES OF CANCER

It is believed that cancer cells arise from normal cells that have undergone a change called *carcinogenesis*. Throughout history there have been various theories as to how the original cancer cell is produced. Recently, researchers have identified and isolated single genes in several types of human cancer called *oncogenes* ("onco" comes from the Greek word *onkos*, meaning "mass" or "tumor"). When introduced into mouse cells, oncogenes have turned them into cancer cells. Many scientists believe that oncogenes are commonly present in our cells, but remain dormant unless "turned on" by carcinogens.

It is natural to wonder why such troublemakers exist in the first place. Scientists believe that oncogenes are somehow involved in normal growth and may be needed at some point in human development—before birth or during childhood—and then are "switched off" when they are no longer needed. Oncogenes, it is believed, become troublemakers only when the chromosomes break and then repair themselves: Sometimes the chromosomes accidentally rearrange themselves and the oncogene is misplaced in the process. If, during repair, the oncogene winds up next to an "active region" on the chromosome, it becomes inadvertently "turned on." Once we know what turns an oncogene on, perhaps we will learn what turns it off. This would open up a whole new area of research that could ultimately lead to a cure for cancer.

The current view also includes the theory that cancer is a two-step process of *initiation* and *promotion*. According to this theory, the initiators prime the cell and so set the stage for cancer development. Initiators include carcinogens such as viruses, radiation, and chemicals such as those contained in toxic waste or food. But these initiated cells are harmless and behave normally and eventually die—they may even be repaired or normalized by the body—unless promoters are also present. Promoters include anything that enhances the effect of an initiator such as diet, hormones, chemicals, environmental conditions, or an inherited predisposition.

This theory looks promising and would help to explain why everyone who smokes doesn't get lung cancer, why all X-ray technicians don't get leukemia, and why a diet of junk food doesn't guarantee the development of gastrointestinal cancer.

HOW CANCER GROWS AND SPREADS

Cancer, as we now understand it, consists of well over one hundred different diseases. These, however, fall into four main categories: carcinomas, lymphomas, leukemias, and sarcomas. *Carcinomas* are the most common—between 85 and 90 percent of all cancers are of this type. They are solid tumors or "lumps" originating in the lining (epithelium) of the organ. Examples are carcinoma of the breast, lung, uterus, intestines, esophagus, stomach, and kidney. *Lymphomas*, cancers of the lymphatic system, add up to 5 percent of all cancers. They cause the spleen and lymph nodes to produce abnormal cells. Lymphomas can cause solid tumors to grow in various parts of the body. *Leukemias* are disseminated (circulating) tumors accounting for 2 percent of cancers. They involve bone marrow, which is the blood-forming system, where they cause abnormal white blood cells to be produced. *Sarcomas*, the rarest form of the four, account for 2 percent of all cancers. These solid tumors develop on the connective tissue of the muscles, bones, nerves, and other organs.

The carcinomas share a common pattern of grown and spread. Cancer of this type begins as a single abnormal cell, which reproduces itself over and over again until it becomes a mass, or a tumor, at which point it can begin to cause problems for the host. If the cancer has spread to other, distant parts of the body, more problems can arise. Nonmalignant tumors are also sometimes called cancers, though they do not spread unless they become malignant. These are not treated with chemotherapy. The medical profession calls all abnormal growths *lesions* or *neoplasms* and precancerous conditions *dysplasia*. The earliest cancer is called *in situ* or *preinvasive cancer*. At this point the cancer is still *localized* and highly curable.

If early cancer goes untreated, it begins to invade the surrounding tissue. Though it is still considered localized, and the cure rates are high, *invasive cancer* is a serious condition. The tumor may grow so large that it crowds out the healthy cells, destroys them, and reduces their functions, or forms an obstruction in a vital pathway of the body, or exerts dangerous pressure on nearby vital organs. Surgical removal of the tumor is usually still possible as a cure, though some or all of the cancerous organ being invaded may be removed as well.

But cancer is not content to grow and grow in one place; at some point during the growth of a tumor, cancer cells begin to break off. They hitch a ride from the bloodstream or the lymphatic system to which they have access, and they circulate freely throughout the body like seeds on the wind. This tendency to spread (metastasize) is perhaps cancer's most frightening and deadliest characteristic. When metastatic or advanced cancer has spread to vital organs such as the brain, bones, liver, or lungs, it cuts off the organ's blood supply or crowds the organ and crushes it. Either way, the organ is no longer able to perform its function. It is not uncommon, for instance, for a woman with metastatic breast cancer to die of liver failure caused by her cancer spreading to that organ. (Even though the cancer is in the liver, it is still breast cancer.)

In general, the longer a tumor exists, the greater the likelihood that it has shed cells, and the greater the number of those cells there will be. It is thought that our immune system is our natural defense against cancer, just as it defends us against other undesirable creatures such as bacteria and viruses. It is widely believed that the immune system controls early cancer cells routinely, before they reproduce to the point where the cancer is large enough to be detected. The immune system may also be able to control advanced cancer, which would explain how the rare but documented "spontaneous remissions" can happen.

But sometimes the immune system slips up, even at the early stage. There are many reasons why it may not successfully destroy the abnormal cells our bodies are constantly churning out, but they all boil down either to a system that is too weak or cancer cells that are too clever. The immune system may be weak because of age, stress, overwhelming systemic infection, factors in the environment, or nutritional deficiencies. Cancer itself may suppress the immune response. There may be a constitutional deficiency. Cancer cells have the unique ability to produce a protective coating that fools the immune system into ignoring them. Unfortunately, surgery, radiation, and chemotherapy—the three major treatments now used against cancer—can also suppress our natural immunity.

Although our immune system may still battle valiantly against proliferating cancer cells, there may eventually be too many of them and our natural defenses become overwhelmed. Our immune system has fumbled the ball, so to speak, and outside treatment now may be called upon to try to save the game.

CHAPTER 2

How Cancer is Treated

In the relatively young field of effective cancer therapy, chemotherapy is still in its infancy. Since no one cancer treatment has proved to be perfect, from the standpoint of either effectiveness or undesirable side effects, chemotherapy is rarely offered as the only treatment. The trend more and more is toward using Combined Modality Therapy—chemo in combination with one or more other forms of therapy, usually the conventional therapies of surgery and radiation, but sometimes along with investigational therapies such as immunotherapy. Recently, aspects of the so-called unorthodox cancer therapies are being taken seriously and integrated into the overall treatment plan.

Though it is a very complex subject when looked at in detail, the fundamentals of chemotherapy are not beyond the grasp of the average person, nor is an understanding of other therapies and how they relate to chemo.

SURGERY

Surgery is the primary treatment for most of the major forms of cancer. However, it is only effective alone as a cure in early, localized solid-tumor cancer. In such cases, the object of the

11

surgery is to physically remove all traces of the malignancy—
to "get it all." When, as in my case, there is evidence or good
reason to believe that the cancer has spread to distant parts of
the body, the object of surgery is to remove as much of the
tumor as possible, and then trust in radiation or chemotherapy
to control or destroy the remaining cells that have escaped the
scalpel. Some experts believe, however, that a tumor begins
to shed cells from the very beginning of its growth, and so
even in "early cancer" there is the possibility of spread. Surgery
may cure cancer in these cases only because few enough cells
were shed for the immune system to handle. Surgery may also
be used to remove metastases in some types of cancer and for
palliation of symptoms such as blockage or pain.

A certain percentage of patients do not survive cancer surgery, and pain is frequently present after the extensive surgery
that cancer often requires. But perhaps most distressing of all
results is the change in body image that surgery leaves in its
wake. Many patients say they feel mutilated or somehow "not
whole" afterward, especially if the affected area is highly visible, useful, or symbolic.

RADIATION THERAPY

Radiation therapy, or radiotherapy, is the recommended primary treatment of choice for some forms of cancer, such as
early Hodgkin's disease, some lung cancers, and head and neck
cancers. It may be used alone for cure, but it is often used in
conjunction with surgery or chemotherapy. Radiation is also
effective as palliation to relieve symptoms of cancer.

The radiotherapy may be administered from outside the body
via special "megavoltage" machines whose radiation penetrates
deep inside the body, avoiding healthy tissue as much as possible. Or it may be internal—a radioactive isotope, encapsu-
lated in a container such as a needle, tube, or seed, is implanted
in the body, either directly into the cancer or nearby. Radio-
isotopes may also be injected into an organ or into the bloodstream, where they go directly to the tumor.

Radiation therapy changes cancer cells' chemistry with rays
or charged particles. When the radiation reaches the tumor
cells, it damages the DNA and makes it impossible for the
present cells or the next generation of cells to reproduce. In
effect, the tumor becomes "sterile."

Radiation has its own set of advantages and drawbacks. Like surgery, this treatment is most effective when it can be used locally. Unlike surgery, it can destroy a tumor without grossly disfiguring the patient; it leaves vital structures intact. It does not work on widely spread metastases unless wide field radiation is used, but this technique has serious side effects on healthy tissue. Cancers vary greatly in their "radiosensitivity": Radiation is highly effective for certain types of cancers, somewhat effective for some, and not at all for others. The tumor must be in a location where the radiation can reach it.

Even with improved technology, some normal tissue does get damaged from radiation. This includes a wide spectrum of side effects: skin reactions such as dryness, itchiness, and burns; loss of hair; lowered energy and appetite; constipation or diarrhea; sore mouth or throat; changes in taste perception; tooth and ear problems; and nausea and vomiting. In addition, radiation has been shown to have the ability to cause leukemia, fertility problems, and birth defects.

CHEMOTHERAPY

You will find a more detailed picture of chemotherapy later in this book; but for now, this quick sketch will help you understand where chemo fits in with the other therapies used to treat cancer.

Chemotherapy literally means the treatment of disease with chemicals, or drugs. Usually, though, the term is understood to mean treatment with anticancer drugs. Of the three major conventional cancer treatments, chemotherapy is the new kid on the block; the post–World War II era is generally considered the beginning of its development. Now about forty drugs are in standard use alone or in many different combinations. In addition, new drugs and new combinations of drugs are constantly being investigated and evaluated, bringing the total up to over one hundred.

Chemotherapy is unique among the conventional approaches to cancer treatment because chemicals have the ability to circulate throughout the body. Only chemicals can reach cancer cells that have broken off solid tumors and spread to distant sites and that may be undetectable and/or untouchable by local treatments; only chemicals are useful in treating disseminated tumors of the blood and lymph. Chemotherapy works because it is *cytotoxic*—it poisons the cells, especially those that reproduce rapidly, as cancer cells do. But as with other therapies, chemo doesn't always work. And because normal cells are also vulnerable to varying degrees, there are also many potential side effects, the most common of which are loss of energy, loss of hair, nausea and vomiting, and susceptibility to infection.

Originally, chemotherapy was used only as a last resort after all else had failed. This tactic has changed drastically. Using chemotherapy as a second line of defense, after a recurrence has already happened, is an approach that has failed to improve the survival of many patients with the most common solid tumors. Chemotherapy is being given earlier and earlier during the course of the disease because as with the other modalities, that is when it works the best. Today, chemotherapy may be the treatment of choice to actually cure certain cancers. But the newest strategy is to use chemotherapy as *adjuvant therapy* as soon as possible right after surgery or radiation "debulked" a tumor or "reduced the tumor burden." It is hoped that when used this way, chemo will prevent or postpone suspected micrometastases from causing a recurrence. Chemotherapy is also being used after surgery to shrink already evident nonoperable metastases. It is sometimes used before surgery to reduce the size of a tumor and make it more operable, or along with radiation to make a tumor more susceptible. Chemotherapy cures some cancers, but not all; however, even when a cure is not achieved, chemo is enabling people to control their cancer for many years and allowing them to live longer than they would have without it. Though inroads are being made in minimizing the side effects, they are still a problem for many people, and whether the risk is worth the benefit is always an individual choice. But as Dr. Oliver Cope writes in his book *The Breast*, "Drugs are our first new hope in twenty-five years."

HORMONE THERAPY

Hormones are substances that are naturally produced by our endocrine glands; their job is to stimulate other organs. If a cancer begins in tissues that are affected by hormones, usually the tumor will be affected by them too. Such tumors are called hormone-sensitive; by changing the hormonal environment we can affect a tumor's growth. In premenopausal women, for example, drugs that suppress hormones may cause a breast tumor to stop growing or to shrink. In postmenopausal women, adding hormones may have the same effect.

Originally, hormone therapy consisted of the surgical removal of the glands that produced the hormones (ablative surgery). This method is still used. But in addition, synthetic hormones or hormone suppressants are often given alone or along with other anticancer drugs for certain types of cancer including cancer of the breast, uterus, prostate, thyroid, kidney, and lymphomas, leukemias, and myelomas. Even though their action is very different from that of the other drugs, hormone therapy is a type of chemotherapy. This field is considered experimental, but it is in fact incorporated into many standard treatments.

Unlike the other drugs used in chemotherapy, hormone therapy is not cytotoxic to cells—it does not kill them directly. These drugs don't cure, but they may cause long-term remissions or enhance the effect of cytotoxic drugs. Their side effects are usually mild compared with those of their more toxic cousins. In addition to their antitumor activity, hormones may be used to reduce certain side effects of chemotherapy, including loss of appetite, and to increase a sense of well-being.

Though hormone therapy is used for several kinds of cancer because of their relatively low numbers and mild side effects, in this book "chemotherapy" and "anticancer drugs" will refer to the cytotoxic group of drugs, except when hormones are specifically mentioned.

INVESTIGATIONAL THERAPIES

Because even the best conventional therapies do not help everyone and have undesirable side effects, studies of new, promising therapies are constantly being conducted under the auspices of the medical mainstream. The new theories and techniques are tried, first on animals and then on humans, to see whether they work better and are less harmful than the techniques currently available. Even the standard therapies so widely used now were once experimental.

Experimental treatments consist mostly of innovations in the three traditional therapies such as new radiation and surgical technologies, new ways of administering chemotherapy, and new chemotherapy drugs or combinations of drugs. Chemotherapy is the freshest example of this; only fifteen years ago it was being given almost exclusively in an experimental setting. In fact, because chemotherapy now offers a chance for survival in many cases of cancer where there was none, this is where most of the investigational trials are being conducted. (See pp. 290–94.)

Another approach to treating cancer that is causing a lot of excitement is that of immunotherapy. Immunotherapy utilizes a whole new category of chemical compounds called "biologic response modifiers" (or "biologicals"). The common goal of these biochemical substances is to punch up the body's defenses—to harness and enhance the body's natural ability to take care of itself.

One branch of immunotherapy involves introducing substances such as bacteria or altered cancer cells that stimulate the body to attack them; in the process, the body's active cancer cells are also attacked.

Another method being developed is to administer antibodies, such as man-made antibodies (*hybridomas* or "antibody factories") and monoclonal antibodies. Though they show some promise when used alone, in the future it may be possible to attach anticancer drugs to these "guided missiles," deliver them directly to the tumor cells, and spare the healthy tissue.

The biological response modifiers also include interferon, a protein found naturally in the body. Interferon first became recognized for its antiviral abilities but soon was hailed for its anticancer properties. Also included in this group is the possible development of drugs that will cause the cancer cells to revert to normal cells, rather than causing their death. Exciting new work is being done with a cancer-destroying substance called *tumor necrosis factor* (TNF), which is found in normal human cells.

This whole approach to cancer treatment is appealing because it appears to be "natural" and the side effects are dissimilar to those of surgery, radiation, and chemotherapy. However, immunology—the most developed of the biologicals—has its own set of possible disturbing side effects including flulike symptoms of chills, fever, nausea, general malaise, and body aches, and seizures, ulcers, and scarring at the site of the injection. In spite of the early brouhaha with which immunology was greeted, biologicals such as interferon have thus far not lived up to expectations. They are not yet the miracle cure for cancer, but they do show exciting potential. For now, they are best used along with standard therapy as complementary treatment. As such, they can enhance its effects or help the body recover from the damage done by these treatments or the disease itself, and prolong a remission or survival time.

Hyperthermia is an approach that is based upon the theory that fever is a key element in our biologic defense against disease. Laboratory tests have shown that heat can stimulate the white blood cells in our immune system to attack cancer cells. It is theorized that heat also sensitizes cancer cells and makes them more vulnerable to radiation or chemotherapy.

Researchers have also been experimenting with ways to tailor chemotherapy treatments to each individual tumor, rather than relying on the drugs' past performance with other people's tumors. For example, drugs may be pretested on the cancer outside the patient's body. A sample of the cancer is taken and the cells are grown in test tubes. Several anticancer drugs are applied to the different groups of cells. The drugs that are most effective against the samples are used on the patient. A variation of this technique utilizes cells grown in specially bred "nude mice." These mice have no hair and no immune systems, and the cells grow in them readily. The nude mice then act as "stand-ins" for the patient.

It is hoped that these techniques will take some of the guesswork out of chemotherapy, thus saving valuable time and needless wear and tear on the patient. Tailoring techniques suffer, however, from great expense; and, it should be added, responses in test tubes or nude mice do not necessarily correlate well with responses in humans.

Bone marrow transplants are very hazardous, complex procedures that are nevertheless being used with greater frequency. The bone marrow, which produces blood cells, can be severely affected when huge amounts of radiation or chemotherapy are given. (These potentially fatal amounts, which attempt to wipe out as much of the diseased marrow as possible, are sometimes the only hope for curing leukemia.) So bone marrow cells— from a twin or biologically compatible sibling—are transplanted in the patient. The healthy marrow replaces the cancerous marrow and in some cases brings about a cure. In other cases, the transplanted cells set up an immunologic reaction that can be fatal. A variation of this procedure is that the bone marrow is taken from the patient while in remission, and this seeks to bypass the possibility of an immune reaction.

Other methods being used experimentally include instilling

drugs into specific body cavities where tumors occur; *chemoembolization*, which enables the drugs to be delivered directly to the tumor and to block off the tumor's blood supply at the same time; and encapsulating drugs in *liposomes*, which dissolve and release the drugs only when exposed to heat, distributing them directly to tumor cells.

It is very important to realize that what you read, hear, or see about cancer "breakthroughs" is usually simplified, exaggerated, and premature. These methods are usually available only to test tubes and laboratory animals, but to few or no people. Dr. Thomas Fahey, who is in charge of the outpatient department at New York City's Memorial Sloan-Kettering, is concerned that "there's a lot of premature media hype about cancer treatment. I think it raises public expectations and sends them off on wild-goose chases."

Dr. Richard Gralla, also at Memorial Sloan-Kettering, agrees that the media do more harm than good:

> "The media look for pop items—whatever they might be—in order to sell a program, to sell the news. A sports announcer knows about sports: If there's a trade in the Yankees to get rid of a leftfielder, the announcer will go into an in-depth analysis of what a bad move that was or what a great move that was. But for the most part, reporters don't know enough about science and appear to be unmotivated to learn more. A responsible reporter shouldn't accept a press release on a breakthrough at face-value. He should call several experts and ask them if they think it's a breakthrough. Most of the time, people will not have very exciting things to say. They'll say, 'Well, we hope so, it'll take a little bit of time.' That's pretty safe, but it also may be fairly accurate, but it's not a 'hot story.'"

UNORTHODOX THERAPIES

Although they may bear a resemblance to investigational therapies, unorthodox cancer therapies (also known as nontraditional, unproven, alternative, nonconventional, or nontoxic therapies), exist for the most part outside the realm of mainstream cancer medicine. Many of these therapies attempt to stimulate the patient's immune system to the point where it is able to control or rid the body of cancer. Rather than treating the symptom (the tumor), they claim to treat the cause (faulty general health). A good proportion of these therapies are based on special diets. In addition, some include nutritional supplements, enzymes, glandular extracts, and other substances and practices designed to detoxify the body, build health, and restore balance. However, not all rely on diet. For example, Lawrence Burton, Ph.D., who treats cancer at his Immunology Researching Centre in Freeport, Grand Bahama Island, calls his therapy "immunoaugmentation," and utilizes blood fractions that are deficient in the cancer patient's blood. Patients undergoing unorthodox therapies are also frequently advised to manage stress through exercise, some form of psychotherapy, mind control, or visualization.

In contrast to surgery, radiation, and chemotherapy, which have side effects because they harm normal tissue, alternative therapies are usually nontoxic, noninvasive, and do not endanger normal tissue. This, combined with their strong holistic philosophy, makes their approach immensely appealing.

The overwhelming problem with unorthodox therapies is that we are not sure about the possibility of benefit because they have not undergone the kind of scientific support and testing that the standard and experimental mainstream-endorsed therapies have received. Unfortunately, almost all the evidence about their effectiveness is anecdotal or testimonial in nature, or remains unpublished by accepted medical journals. The medical mainstream says this lack of concrete proof of efficacy is why it does not recommend these treatments to its cancer patients as primary treatments. Although the direct risk is attractively low, many doctors feel they are indirectly harmful because patients who go for alternative therapy are lured away from effective traditional treatment, and possibly a cure.

Patients who are attracted to alternative therapies have nowhere to turn for objective views. (Some proponents of these therapies are listed in the Appendix.) Your oncologist should, however, at least try to answer any questions you may have and be willing to discuss the issue calmly. The social service department or dietary department of your hospital is another potential source for information. Though it is a subject that is being brought up more and more frequently, some patients may still be afraid to bring up unorthodox therapies to their orthodox health practitioners. It is, however, part of their jobs to be informed and to help you become informed in order to make

an intelligent decision—one that is right for you. And it is
your right and responsibility to still any doubts you might have
about your therapy.

COMBINING THERAPIES

In modern cancer care it is becoming rare to use only one
type, or modality, of treatment. Today a combination of two
or more is increasingly favored, because one enhances the effect
of another or supplies a therapeutic strength where the others
are weak. Though the three standard therapies—surgery, radiation, and chemotherapy—are the most often combined, cancer care providers and their patients are dipping also into the
investigational or "unproven" therapies with greater frequency,
which enables them to enjoy the benefits of both and spares
them the agony of making an either/or decision.

It is becoming clear that all nontraditional therapies cannot
forever be dismissed as completely worthless in light of continuing revelations about the interrelationship of the immune
system, the mind, nutrition, and cancer. As a result, some
practicing oncologists are beginning to suggest—or at least not
object to—a more "holistic" approach for their patients
undergoing traditional therapies. Some elements of the alternative approach such as relaxation, visualization, immunology,
and nutritional therapy are being used in conjunction with standard therapies such as chemotherapy. There are even formal
investigations being conducted, for example, of thymosin—a
hormone produced by the thymus gland, which is the master
gland of the immune system. (Thymosin has for years been
available in the thymus gland extract sold in health food stores.)
Early studies of two traditional Chinese herbal medicines showed
improved immune response and may prove valuable in combination with chemotherapy. There has also been encouraging
work done with bacterial vaccines based on Coley's toxins, a
therapy that had been written off by the American Cancer
Society when it was placed on their "unproven" remedies list,
but that is being used experimentally along with chemo.

In addition, some of the alternative practitioners are soften-
ing their stances and adding either chemotherapy or other traditional treatments to their nontoxic programs, or referring their
patients to mainstream doctors for conventional treatment.

Clearly, there is as yet no single "magic bullet" against cancer, and the best approach seems to be an eclectic one.

Perhaps the most persuasvie argument for opening up the traditional treatment plan to some elements of the alternative therapies does not rest directly on any claims to their possible anticancer abilities. It lies rather in the fact that some of these practices do foster better overall health, help minimize side effects of cancer and chemotherapy, and allow patients to participate more actively in their treatment and assume some control over some aspects of their lives. In a medical world that consists largely of our passively waiting around for people in white coats to pump us full of toxic chemicals, doing health-building things for ourselves, preferably under the guidance of a qualified but accessible professional, is a welcome change. (See Chapters 7–9.)

In the June 17, 1982, issue of the *New England Journal of Medicine*, Barrie R. Cassileth, Ph.D., of the University of Pennsylvania Cancer Center, addressed her colleagues:

"The anti-medicine, pro–self-help bias of the new alternative treatments arises in the context of increasing mistrust and dissatisfaction with the standard healthcare system and with researchers' failure to cure malignant disease. Traditional multimodality care of cancer, often fragmented and associated with a passive role for the patient, contrasts starkly with the active, personalized, nontoxic, home-based alternatives . . . There is something to be learned from the seductive draw of alternative remedies. We may not wish to recommend wheatgrass therapy or spiritual healing in lieu of chemotherapy, but we might well consider the merits of patients' needs for involvement in their own care, their interest in helping themselves through attention to diet, their requirements for personalized attention to self as opposed to disease."

CHAPTER 3

Understanding Chemotherapy

HOW CHEMOTHERAPY BEGAN

Cancer chemotherapy is part of a long medical tradition of using chemical compounds to treat disease. From natural herbs to sophisticated man-made substances, effective medicines were usually discovered accidentally and chemo is no exception.

The lucky accident that made modern cancer chemotherapy possible occurred in 1942, ironically due to a war in which millions of people were killed. In that year, a U.S. naval vessel sank while in the Naples harbor. When the mustard gas it was carrying exploded, the casualties who had been exposed to the poisonous gas were examined and it was found that large numbers of the cells in their bone marrow had disappeared and their lymphatic systems had atrophied. The significance of this was not lost on C. P. "Dusty" Rhodes, the chief of the biological branch of the U.S. Army Chemical Warfare Service, who was on leave from Memorial Hospital Cancer Center where he was the director. He began large-scale testing on animals of hundreds of drugs similar to the poisonous gas that went down with the ship. These were found to inhibit lymphoid tumors in the animals. The drugs were tested on humans with Hodgkin's disease in 1943, and the subjects experienced temporary remissions.

22

Around the same time that the beneficial effects of nitrogen mustard (mustard gas) were so serendipitously discovered, scientists began to realize they had reached an impasse in cancer treatment. Surgery and radiation were local treatments, inappropriate for systemic, disseminated cancers of and by the blood and lymph systems, and ineffective once solid tumors had visibly spread. But more frustrating was the fact that these treatments didn't always cure what appeared to be localized cancer. Scientists theorized, and proved in experiments, that even one or a few surviving cancer cells could result in a recurrence.

Because the preliminary results of the early cancer drugs were so promising, a large-scale search for other drugs that were effective against cancer was begun. In 1955 the National Cancer Institute, an arm of the National Institutes of Health, directed a mammoth screening program. Investigators in England, continental Europe, and Japan participated. Hundreds of thousands of drugs were tested, with 40,000 as the all-time high in 1975. This screening continues today, albeit on a more organized, and smaller, scale. (See pp. 290–94.)

HOW CHEMOTHERAPY WORKS

Chemotherapy is the only scientifically proven method we have that can reach virtually every part of the body to seek and destroy cancer cells that surgery and radiation can't reach, and that even sensitive instruments can't see. It is able to penetrate every nook and cranny because it circulates throughout the body just the way the cancer cells do by flowing through the bloodstream. Once the drug meets up with a cancer cell, it wreaks havoc in a number of ways, which are only partly understood.

Chemotherapy affects the course of cancer by taking advantage of the cancer cell's penchant for constant reproduction. Almost all the drugs used in chemotherapy suppress cancer by somehow altering the cells' DNA and thus their ability to reproduce. Since DNA is most vulnerable to drug interference during the reproductive phases of the life cycle, cancer cells are more likely to be affected than the bulk of the body's normal cells which reproduce at a much more relaxed pace. Thus, the very characteristic that makes cancer so dangerous has proved to contribute to its undoing. In scientific terminology, chemotherapy drugs are either "cell-cycle specific" (lethal to cells only during a specific reproductive phase) or "cell-cycle non-specific" (able to sabotage the cells no matter what phase they are in). Dr. Ronald Bash, an oncologist at the Albert Einstein Hospital in the Bronx explains it this way: "In a sense, the inner workings of cells (cancerous and otherwise) are like gear-boxes; what chemotherapy does is to throw a biochemical monkey wrench into the gearbox causing the machine to grind to a halt—causing the cells to stop working, to die."

WHEN CHEMOTHERAPY DOESN'T WORK

If chemotherapy works at all, you might wonder why it doesn't work all the time. No medicines, not even those for minor ailments, work all the time. Though cancer is admittedly far more complex than athlete's foot, pimples, and headaches, it may be a bit unrealistic to expect a science that has failed to produce surefire cures for these relatively simple conditions to be able consistently to crack a sophisticated disease like cancer. Since cancer is not a foreign invader like bacteria, but an aberration of the body's own cells, it is in fact amazing that anticancer drugs work at all.

The reasons chemotherapy may fail are legion. First of all, there may simply be too many cancer cells, growing too rapidly, for the drugs to wipe out or even keep at bay. If the goal is to cure, every single cancer cell must die. If even one cell is left behind, and manages to proliferate, the cancer will recur.

Chemotherapy may fail because it works best when there are (a) small numbers of cancer cells that are (b) actively dividing. These conditions are not always present when chemotherapy is given. In "cell kinetics" experiments, it has been shown that drugs destroy a constant fraction or percentage of cells, not a constant number. So if there are 10 trillion cancer cells and 99 percent are killed, 100 billion are still left after the first treatment! After the second treatment, 1 billion cells are left, and after the third, 10 million remain. The proportion of cells killed is the same, but each time a smaller number of cells is killed. The cells that are resting rather than actively reproducing escape the drugs' killing effects. In between treatments, when it is safe, the resting cells resume production and replace the ones that have been killed. Chemotherapy under

the best of conditions is a matter of taking two steps forward
and one step backward, and it is very difficult to make enough
progress to kill off every single cell.

Kinetic studies have also shown that as the cancer increases
in size—the more cells it contains—the number of actively
reproducing cells (the "growth fraction") decreases. The higher
the number you start with, the harder and longer you have to
work at getting the cell population down, because not only are
there more cells to kill, there are more cells that are not vulnerable.

In addition, the tumor may not be getting enough of the
drug to affect it. Once a drug is injected or ingested, it becomes
extremely diluted and weak because it is distributed throughout
the bloodstream and tissues of the body. Many tumors do not
have a robust blood supply, so drugs may not reach them. In
addition, it has been problematic in getting drugs at all to the
brain and central nervous system because there is a natural
protective mechanism called the blood-brain barrier, which prevents drugs from passing through, though there are now ways
of getting around this.

Time works against chemotherapy. The body quickly begins
to break down toxic substances such as chemotherapy drugs
into less harmful substances—another protective mechanism—and then excretes them. Cancer cells and normal cells
alike can therefore be exposed to the drugs for just a minimum
amount of time—minutes. Since many drugs work on cells
only during a specific phase of their reproductive cycle, only
those cells that happen to be in the vulnerable phase will be
affected during the few minutes that the drug is viable. Cells
in other cycles escape unscathed.

Because the drugs are also highly toxic to normal cells, we
are limited in the amounts of the drugs we can tolerate, and it
is said that chemotherapy drugs have a low "therapeutic index."
The difference in the amount needed to kill more cancer cells
than healthy cells is low; sometimes it is zero. Many promising
drugs never get off the drawing board because the amount that
would totally wipe out a tumor would also kill the patient.

Third, there is the possibility of drug resistance. A single
tumor is usually heterogeneous (composed of a mixture of
different cells). Each type of cell varies in its ability to metastasize, in its susceptibility to drugs, and in its other properties. It is thought that the older a tumor is, the more likely
it is to be heterogeneous, thus increasing the probability that

some of the cells will be resistant to drugs. In addition, resistance develops as the treatment progresses—just as insects, bacteria, and other unwanted creatures adapt and become less sensitive to pesticides and antibiotics. Eventually all the sensitive cells may be killed, but the sturdy ones remain and continue to grow. There is new, chilling evidence that indicates that the very things that kill most patients—metastases—do not arise from the random survival of cells released from the primary tumor, as was previously thought. Rather, they are growths of special tumor cells that are particularly heterogeneous, clever, and resistant to the body's own defenses as well as to drugs. It is as if the parent tumor sends its brightest, most athletic children out into the world of the cancer patient's body.

These are the main reasons why chemotherapy is more effective the earlier it is used, and after the bulk of the tumor has been reduced by surgery or radiation. They help explain why chemotherapy doesn't always work, and why it sometimes works only a little bit, for a little while. (And why cancer has been compared to crabgrass!)

CHAPTER 4

Getting the Best Care

It is the rare cancer patient who doesn't get thrown into a panic after the initial diagnosis, who can think clearly and doesn't feel rushed into treatment, who feels well enough to be able to explore treatment possibilities. It is natural to feel overwhelmed and to want to trust and rely on the first doctor you see. But in most cases of cancer, it is not dangerous to take a few weeks to digest the new earth-shattering information. On the contrary, since the quality of chemotherapy varies so greatly, it is wise to take steps to see that you get the correct diagnosis and the best treatment. The quality and quantity of your life depend on it. A little effort now can make a big difference later on.

The single most important step you can take is to see at least one qualified cancer specialist. Only then is it possible to get a firm, detailed diagnosis and clear picture of your options. The final step is to evaluate the doctor(s) and treatment(s) and choose whichever suits you individually.

WHY A CANCER SPECIALIST (ONCOLOGIST)?

Most often, suspicion of cancer or the initial diagnosis comes from a family doctor or a specialist in the area in which symptoms are first noted, such as a gynecologist for a breast lump or a urologist for a testicular or prostate problem. These physicians may be very qualified in their particular fields and may have treated cancer years ago. However, in most cases, they are not the best qualified to treat cancer today. Because cancer diagnosis and treatment has become so complex, a special branch of medicine called "oncology" has evolved. Oncology (from the Greek *onkos* meaning "lump" and *logos* meaning "study") is a branch of medicine that deals specifically with the study of tumors. A doctor who is specially trained in this field is called an *oncologist*.

Today there are surgical oncologists, radiation oncologists, and medical oncologists (chemotherapists), any and all of whom may be involved in your overall treatment plan. Oncologists usually refer patients to their colleagues in the other subspecialties when they feel a multidisciplinary approach would be beneficial. For instance, a surgical oncologist may refer a patient to a medical oncologist for chemotherapy. My own experience followed this familiar pattern: My gynecologist examined my breast lump and sent me to a surgical oncologist who specialized in treating breast disease; my surgeon then suggested that I see a medical oncologist for further treatment.

Whereas your primary concern is your chemotherapist, it is to your advantage if all the members of your treatment team are well qualified. The best oncologists are usually board-eligible or board-certified, meaning they have been formally trained in this subspecialty and, if certified, have passed an exam.

Your surgeon, therefore, should be board-certified and specialize in your type of cancer. If radiotherapy is on the agenda, you should go to a board-certified radiation oncologist—rather than to a radiologist whose training is mostly in diagnosis.

And anyone who has been told that he or she needs chemotherapy should be seen by a board-certified or board-eligible medical oncologist, who has received two years of formal training in the use of chemotherapeutic drugs.

Hematologists—internists with special training in the area of blood—were the first to use chemotherapy because the earliest cancers treated with drugs were the "blood cancers." Board-certified or board-eligible hematologists with training and experience in cancer still treat the disease. Though they may continue to confine themselves to blood cancers (leukemias, lymphomas, and myelomas), many also treat other cancers. More recently, board-certified internists who are not hematologists have begun specializing in chemotherapy.

The importance of being seen by at least one qualified medical oncologist cannot be overemphasized. Dr. Ronald Bash, a hematologist/oncologist at the Albert Einstein Hospital in the Bronx, says: "There are a lot of people giving chemotherapy who probably shouldn't. Some surgeons, for example, particularly for colon and breast cancer. I've gotten patients who have had adjuvant chemotherapy for colon cancer which has been shown to be useless, or very close to useless."

Chemotherapeutic drugs are highly toxic and the treatment can be very complex. Their use changes rapidly, and the prescribing doctor must not only know of their availability, he must know how to use them and how to monitor the patient properly to achieve the ultimate therapeutic effect without severe toxicity. Only a physician who specializes in the use of these drugs is qualified to evaluate a cancer, to choose a chemotherapy protocol, and in most cases, to administer the drugs. If you like, you can still be seen by your primary physician during your cancer treatment and sometimes even receive some portion of your treatment from him, provided it is under the guidance of an oncologist.

WHERE TO FIND AN ONCOLOGIST

Comprehensive cancer centers, university hospitals, large medical centers, clinics, community hospitals, and oncologists in private practice all offer chemotherapy. If your primary physician has not referred you to an oncologist, ask him or her for a recommendation, or locate a cancer specialist through another doctor you know, your friends or relatives, the local medical society, the National Cancer Institute (NCI), or the American Cancer Society. You can also contact a hospital directly.

In deciding upon which of these facilities is best for you, getting the best *treatment* should not be confused with getting the best overall *care*; it is possible to get the most effective, up-to-date technical treatment while other needs go unheeded or unfulfilled. For example, some believe a big cancer center is the place for the seriously ill, but others will argue eloquently that these are the very people who should stay closer to home and family. Factors you will need to consider are medical (Which offers the most effective program?), practical (How far am I willing to travel for treatment? How much can I pay?), and personal (Do I like the environment? Do I have a good relationship with the doctor?). The effectiveness of the treatments, the personalities of the doctors, the surroundings in which the treatment is administered, and the cost can and do vary greatly. So does the distance you can travel—be it within your own town, to the next big city, or all the way to another state. Fortunately, most chemotherapy is given on an outpatient basis— only the heaviest doses of the most toxic drugs, and some highly experimental treatments, require hospitalization.

It is a common prejudice that the best place to go for cancer treatment is a big cancer center or university hospital. That is where the famous cancer specialists are, where the most modern technology is available, and where the latest experimental therapies are developed and administered. Yet few people understand what they are or what they have to offer. There are presently twenty-four "comprehensive cancer centers" in this country. This is a special designation given by the National Cancer Institute to cancer centers that have met certain strict, specific criteria. "Clinical cancer centers" are similar to comprehensive cancer centers in many ways, but they do not have the same status.

At one time, cancer centers *did* offer the very best cancer treatment across the board. However, this is no longer necessarily true. Most cancer patients can get just as good chemotherapy—even investigational drugs—much closer to home. The comprehensive cancer centers are the first to admit this.

Linda James, planning analyst in the Department of Strategic Planning which was responsible for the new outpatient chemotherapy unit at Memorial Sloan-Kettering in New York City, notes:

"Hundreds of physicians pass through cancer centers like Memorial each year to train in oncology and then go out all over the country. We screen patients who call to determine whether they really need to come here or can be diagnosed and treated closer to home. Patients may come in for a diagnosis and we may develop and assign a chemotherapy protocol, but then we try to make every effort to locate local physicians and facilities where they can get high-quality treatment."

Dr. Richard Gralla, also at Memorial, offers these guidelines to anyone contemplating going to a comprehensive cancer center. "I would say that people who should come into a cancer center are people with unusual diseases, or people who need a treatment that cannot be offered at another facility."

Dr. James A. Neidhart, chairman of the Department of Medical Oncology at the University of Texas System Cancer Center, M.D. Anderson Hospital and Tumor Institute, states: "My bias is that the research treatment programs at most comprehensive cancer centers or at most clinical cancer centers are probably at least state-of-the-art, or hopefully on the cutting edge. But there's no reason for a person to truck to Columbus, Ohio, or to the Mayo Clinic if there is a good local treatment group that's working with good clinical research programs."

Dr. Michael Van Scoy-Mosher, an oncologist at Cedars-Sinai Medical Center in Los Angeles, says:

"I personally think that the most personalized care is in a private office. I may be prejudiced, but I've spent six years at three different cancer centers, so I do have a basis for comparison. A patient may be sent to a center for a consultation, but he may be seen and evaluated by an intern. At the very end, the attending physician may only briefly see the patient. What value is that? Mostly there's a difference in orientation. The private practitioner should be concerned only with the patient sitting in the room with him. In a cancer center, there is concern for today's patient, but there is just as much concern with the research that will help the patient who will show up five or six years later. That's fine, but I don't want to be that patient sitting in the room today. It's not the way I would want to be treated, and it's not the way I'd want my mother to be treated. However, certain patients really feel confident only if they are treated in a 'Cancer Center.' If I perceive this to be the case, I will recommend a referral there."

Cancer centers have physicians and teams who subspecialize in particular cancers. In certain cases it may be wise for you to contact a cancer center to confirm a complicated diagnosis or to get a second opinion about the treatment of choice. It might also be advantageous for you to begin your treatment at a cancer center, particularly if you require specialized surgery, radiation, or treatment with the latest technical equipment not available at your local hospital. If you are a patient with an unusual or difficult cancer, and for whom the standard or the locally available investigational treatment leaves much to be desired, it may definitely be worthwhile for you to travel to see highly experienced specialists, or to get into a highly experimental investigational program that offers a more promising result.

Another valid reason for seeking treatment at a cancer center is when it is the only source for a particular experimental program that might help you. Your local physician can easily find this out through a new computerized cancer information service called Physicians' Data Query (PDQ), which is available through MEDLARS, the National Library of Medicine's data base subscribed to by hospitals, cancer centers, and medical libraries. This program provides physicians in communities all over the United States with up-to-date information about NCI-supported clinical trials and treatments available in cancer centers, and state-of-the-art cancer treatment information tailored to fit a patient's particular type of cancer; it also allows physicians to direct their patients to board-certified specialists in their geographic regions.

However, cancer centers are not the only source for all investigational protocols—just for the highly experimental ones. The NCI and the cancer centers are trying very hard to see that the public has greater access to the clinical research advances possible only through participating in investigational trials. Regional cooperative oncology groups and the newer Community Clinical Oncology Program (CCOP), established in 1983, allow more patients to enter clinical studies in their own communities. There are no studies that compare the quality of chemotherapy treatments across the board between cancer centers and local facilities.

But there was a reassuring study that compared the results of the Eastern Cooperative Oncology Group consisting of university hospitals or major treatment centers with 100 affiliates consisting of small community hospitals and private-practice groups of physicians. The study involved 97 randomized trials and 4,506 patients. The authors of the report of the study, published in the May 6, 1982, issue of the *New England Journal of Medicine*, wrote that "over a wide spectrum of studies and sites, the survival, response, toxicity, and data quality were the same in affiliates as in major treatment centers."

University hospitals and large medical centers can offer the same advantages as comprehensive cancer centers: up-to-date experimental treatment by highly experienced cancer specialists, and a full range of on-site support services such as blood transfusions, laboratory testing, and social services. They also have many of the same disadvantages of being treated away from home and all that that entails: commuting long distances, which is disruptive and lonely, and possibly uncomfortable and depressing; the hassle and expense of making travel arrangements and perhaps accommodations for outpatients and/or accompanying family; and surroundings that are strange and frightening.

Finally, some patients in large facilities complain that the surroundings are too cold and clinical, that the care is on the impersonal side, that they feel like cancer case #342, with outpatients being seen more by the nurses than by the doctors, and inpatients being seen by a number of different doctors including experienced residents, interns, or students. Dr. Thomas Fahey, deputy chief medical officer of Memorial Sloan-Kettering in New York City, comments on this. "To me, when you talk about support for the chemotherapy patient, it begins when you give the treatment. The environment is important. Our old environment, frankly, was terrible. It was designed fifteen years ago when nobody really thought about it. Now we have a unit that is being designed from the ground up."

Medical clinics generally provide more personal care than do the large cancer centers and hospitals. They often have excellent specialists and offer experimental programs for cancer treatment if these can be given on an outpatient basis. However, back-up services may not be as handy.

Community hospitals often supply excellent care for the average cancer patient. The faces seem friendlier, the care more personalized. Some people are more secure being treated at smaller hospitals where they feel there is more compassion, more respect for their wishes, and less risk of becoming guinea pigs or being lost in the shuffle. However, some feel that small hospitals, especially privately owned ones, are more likely to have limited or substandard services. They may not offer the treatment plan you need, although they can often follow through with a chemotherapy protocol that has been established by more experienced specialists at larger hospitals, medical centers, or cancer centers. In most cases, adults can be treated in an accredited community hospital under experienced direction.

Medical oncologists in private practice can give you highly personalized care in relatively small, unthreatening, comfortable surroundings. Sometimes they can be more than comfortable. My oncologist has his practice in a lovely brick town house. The office is furnished just like a real home—carpet, wallpaper, sofas, chairs, even chamber music tapes that play continually—and has a lovely garden I could gaze upon before and during my treatment. It was very comfortable and that made me feel more at ease than a run-of-the-mill doctor's office would have.

Some physicians have a private practice in a hospital, and full and immediate access to back-up services. Some patients feel safer with physicians in a group practice or in a hospital because this means they are subject to constant review by their peers. At any rate, an oncologist should be affiliated with an accredited hospital in case a patient needs to be admitted. One that was trained at a cancer center and retains his or her ties is more likely to provide up-to-date treatment; private physicians often consult with their fellow specialists at a cancer center and follow through on a treatment program initiated there.

It makes very little sense, then, for the majority of cancer patients to travel very far from home for their chemotherapy treatments. This should come as a relief if you are one of the 80 percent of all cancer patients who are treated in their communities: You are not necessarily getting treatment that is inferior to the treatment you would receive at a large cancer center. And you have the advantage of keeping the disruption of your life to a minimum. (As one health professional asserted, "Patients will do anything to be able to go home at night.") It cannot be stressed enough, however, that you be treated by a competent medical oncologist, and not a local physician who does not specialize in this field.

EVALUATING YOUR ONCOLOGIST

Cancer is a frightening disease that may require treatment or monitoring for the rest of your life. The kind of relationship you have with your oncologist can exert a large influence upon the way you feel about your disease and its treatment. I was very resistant to the idea of having chemotherapy at first. But I found a wonderful oncologist who trained at a comprehensive cancer center and who was kind, open to questions, spoke regular English (not medicalese), and even had a sense of humor. I trusted and liked him and that made the therapy less scary to start and more bearable as it wore on.

The ideal is to find a crackerjack oncologist who really knows his stuff *and* who treats you like a human being. It is advisable to ask yourself whether your doctor has the unique combination of good credentials, a compatible personality and approach, and the willingness to answer questions. Is he or she a doctor you will be able to stand seeing every week, or every two weeks, or every month for the duration of your therapy? A doctor you will be able to forgive for making you so miserable with such regularity? Good credentials are no guarantee that the doctor will treat the person as well as the disease, that you will get the best treatment and overall care.

In his book, *The Facts About Cancer*, Charles F. McKhann describes the special relationship a cancer patient has with the oncologist:

> "It is a long-term association that should sustain you through good and bad, through the uncertainties of the disease, the triumphs of success, or the disappointment of unsuccessful treatment, possibly to the very end of life. A doctor in whom you have real confidence can make everything more tolerable. Your doctor should be compassionate, understanding, and interested in you as a person as well as a patient. If honesty is important to you, insist that you discuss your disease and its treatment openly. For many, however, it is more important to know that the lines of communication are open and that your questions will be answered than to ask actual questions at the time. While it is not essential for good care, it helps a lot to have a doctor whom you really like."

Other pluses to look for are a cheerful, pleasant office, twenty-four-hour phone accessibility, laboratory diagnostic tools such as X-ray and blood testing nearby or in the office.

Most patients would agree with this portrait of the ideal doctor-patient relationship. I know that the relationship I had with my oncologist shaped my attitude and ability to cope. While I was researching this book, my heart went out to patients who said their oncologists fell far short of the mark. Many complained about a coldness, a lack of communication and information, a lack of respect and concern; about doctors who seem too busy, who use technical language, or who keep patients waiting very long times without apology or explanation. These failings add insult to injury; chemotherapy is enough of a strain without oncologists adding to their patients' difficulties, as these patients attest:

> "I have a theory that all oncologists are Serbo-Croatian terrorists-in-training just waiting to get their terrorist licenses and practicing medicine in the meantime. They are so single-minded in their ruthless pursuit of knowledge; they strike me more as scientists doing battle than as caring professionals."

> "I hate the patronizing attitude doctors have toward women. I wonder how much oncologists really listen to their patients."

> "The man had no bedside manner. There was only one reason I stayed with him: I had been told he was a big man in his field and the best in the city."

Although an overly technical approach and lack of human warmth has been a charge leveled at the medical profession in general, there seems to be widespread agreement among patients and doctors alike that there is a unique "oncology personality."

Dr. William Grace, chief of oncology at St. Vincent's Hospital in New York City, says:

> "Oncologists can be a funny breed. Many can be highly intellectual, cold, and terribly austere. They can be rather abrasive and not quite so personable. This may be due to the fact that they are involved in an emotionally stressful field for a long period of time."

Dr. Ronald Bash adds:

"Communicating with patients is an art and some oncologists can't do it. Sometimes it's a question of doctors lapsing into medical jargon. Most patients don't understand it, and it builds a little barrier between them and their doctors, of which most doctors are unaware.

"If you don't talk to your patients, you can insulate yourself from their pain. But I think part of the 'territory' is accepting the fact that a number of your patients are going to suffer. You have to learn to endure it, too. The justification that some physicians make for their distant attitude is that if you don't achieve that distance, you end up getting very nuts. That's only partly true at best."

My oncologist says he feels "a tremendous outrage" on the behalf of cancer patients:

"It's a chilling disease. Almost all individuals who have it are inclined to feel shut out from the rest of the world, and to a large extent they are. And because of its nature, taking care of dying patients tends to have a chilling effect on the doctor. It is very easy to be very cold and unable to hear about the aspects of life that are difficult. It's extremely important for the oncologist to be available and willing to hear about that aspect of human existence. There are other people to whom the patient can talk, but it's difficult if the doctor is just writing the prescription and coldly looking at the size of the tumor."

Many experienced patients and professionals point out the importance of entering into a partnership with your oncologist in which you regard each other as equals. They also believe that being reasonably knowledgeable about cancer and its treatment is an intrinsic part of coping. It is our right and responsibility to be active, informed participants in the vital decisions affecting our bodies. The more we know, the less of the unknown there is to fear and the better partners we make in the treatment process, because we meet our doctors on more equal footing. And as our understanding about the potentials and limitations of oncology improves, so will our relations with our doctors improve.

A satisfactory relationship between you and your oncologist can make any chemotherapy plan go more easily and the continual followup more pleasant. Honesty, compatability, mutual respect, an openness and willingness to communicate, trust, confidence—these are the characteristics of any good relationship. They are difficult but not impossible to attain, provided that both parties are aware of their importance and are willing to encourage each other to cultivate them.

IS CHEMOTHERAPY FOR YOU?

Patients usually regard undertaking chemotherapy with *at least* some ambivalence and fear. Having a clear, realistic picture of its goals, the costs versus the benefits, and your alternatives will help you avoid either a distortedly negative picture that might lead to a refusal of beneficial treatment, or an overly optimistic or naïve one that may lead you to accept a treatment you decide is ultimately not worth it to you and may lead to disappointment and resentment.

Dr. Michael Van Scoy-Mosher emphasizes:

"Chemotherapy is a true cooperative venture. The physician gives the drugs, but the real work is done by the patient. As much as I might sympathize, it is the patient who undergoes the unpleasant therapy. I think whatever it takes—seeing five different doctors, reading in libraries, talking to other people—it's very important that they become convinced that they have made the right decision.

"A lot of the bad things you hear about chemotherapy occur because of the ways it's been misused, such as giving chemotherapy to people whom there's no chance in the world that chemotherapy is going to help—give them chemotherapy for a couple of months, make them bald, make them sicker, and they die anyway. You know what the family of the patient says later? 'That chemotherapy—it's the worst thing in the world. It killed my brother—he was bald, he was sick.' It's hard to separate out the effects of the cancer from those of chemotherapy anyway, but the next time someone in that family gets cancer, they say they will never take chemotherapy. So I have to undo all of that if they've had a previous experience."

These patients bear him out:

"I had a fear of chemo. I knew people who had had it, and I had seen the horrors of chemo. They just faded away, they became skeletons. But now I realize that there's chemo, and then there's chemo. I just thought everybody got the same thing and reacted the same way."

"I didn't like the idea that they were going to be putting poison in my system. I was upset about losing my hair—all my life it's been my pride. I had already had gum problems and now they were telling me I might have mouth sores. As soon as the doctor left the room, I had this terrific outburst of crying. I cried and cried and really got it out of my system. And then I started to get hold of myself. If I didn't have it, and God forbid something happens a few years from now, I'm going to say to myself, 'you know you had a shot at this and you didn't take it.' It took me forty-five minutes to decide that I was going to take the best shot I had."

Others accept their doctor's advice without question, without finding out what they are getting into:

"My regular medical GP, the surgeon, and the oncologist had a conference and decided I should have chemo. I was kind of stupid in a way. When they suggested I have it, I said, 'Oh sure,' not knowing what chemo was like. I knew nothing about it. I figured if other people have gone through it, it can't be that bad."

The decision to undergo chemotherapy cannot be made intelligently, confidently, and wholeheartedly unless you have gathered enough pertinent information to allow you to assess the risks versus the benefits for *you*, in your particular circumstances. Your doctor is your *primary* source for medical information and advice. But it should not be left up to him to make the final decision—or to provide all the information you might need in order to make the choice. Dr. Van Scoy-Mosher, for instance, finds:

"In very controversial uses of chemotherapy some patients want me to make the decision for them. Much as they try to pin me down, I won't do it. All I can do is spell out the arguments for and against a treatment. Often they'll leave the office more anxious than when they came in; but the important issue to me is that they've made their own decisions. And in the long run, patients who have made their own decisions do quite well with those decisions. I know that a year or two from then, they'll feel good about it."

His colleague Dr. Richard Gralla says:

"For me, I have to talk to my patients a little bit to find out what their outlook is. I have to tell them what we have available and what their alternatives are. I can give my advice, what I would do if I were they. But ultimately the choice comes to them. Some people say, 'I want this treatment if it's a one in a thousand chance.' Some people say that a three out of four chance of benefit is not good enough. But that's their individual philosophy. I can just tell them their alternatives and help them make that decision.

"What's really important is that people have to understand that when a cure is not possible, then improvement of quality of life becomes a major goal. Some people say they want their quality of life, not their length of life necessarily, to be improved. Usually the two go hand in hand. It is rare to get one without the other, and I think a lot of people don't realize that. If you have improvement in time, usually you have improvement in quality of life during that time."

THE GOALS OF CHEMOTHERAPY

In the early days, chemotherapy was considered a last resort to be used only in terminal cases when all else had failed to cure a cancer. When used so late in the disease, there was every reason for pessimism, for the chances were indeed slim that drugs—or anything—could save anyone at the eleventh hour. Chemotherapy then was highly experimental, and there were relatively few drugs to experiment with. No wonder it usually failed to perform the hoped-for miracles that surgery and radiation had also failed to perform, and it was said that the treatment was worse than the disease.

Although, as my oncologist admits, "Chemotherapy is still in the Stone Age," new drugs have been introduced and we are learning more and more about these drugs and the diseases they treat. We know more about how and when to administer them, how much of them to give, in what combinations, for how long, what side effects to expect and what to do about them, and what kind of response to expect. For instance, we now know that chemotherapy works best when used as early as possible, when the tumor burden is small. The increasing success of chemotherapy is due in large part to the big push toward giving it much sooner than was previously thought advisable, even when there is no detectable spread. However, there are also drugs that are highly effective even in the more advanced, metastatic cancers.

Today, chemotherapy is being used to achieve goals that are both more optimistic and realistic than those in the past. It is being used to cure some cancers outright; to induce long-term remissions in others; to decrease the likelihood of a recurrence or spread after surgery or radiation (adjuvant chemotherapy) in potentially curable cancers; to slow the growth and alleviate symptoms such as pain (palliation) in incurable or recurrent cancers; and to shrink large tumors to operable size and to make radiation more effective.

According to the lastest National Cancer Institute report (November 1983), the overall cancer survival rate for "serious" forms of cancer is 48 percent. The survival rate used is the "relative survival rate"—the percentage of people who can expect to reach the five-year mark or are curable. This rate has been adjusted to take normal life expectancy into consideration and to factor in deaths from other causes such as heart disease and accidents. "Nonserious" cancers—nonmelanoma skin cancer and in situ cervical cancer—are highly curable and are not included.

Dr. Vincent DeVita, head of the NCI, presented a keynote address at the American Cancer Society National Conference held in June 1982. Based on treatments that were available in 1977, he gave these estimated figures about the effectiveness of specific cancer treatments. (These figures are expected to be higher when the effects of the currently available therapies are documented statistically.) Most of the people being cured of cancer each year—220,000—are treated successfully with surgery alone. Of the rest, 90,000 are successfully treated with radiation alone or in combination with surgery. The remaining 46,000 are cured thanks to chemotherapy, either used alone or added to other therapies.

Of the estimated 200,000 people who have chemo each year, 23 percent are cured, and a total of 67 percent derive some benefit from the therapy. Of those who are not cured, 25,000 remain tumor-free for an average of two years, and 63,000 can expect to live one year longer. Although they are being disputed by some, these figures indicate that chemotherapy helps the overwhelming majority of those who have it, and these are people who had very little hope for successful treatment at all.

TO CURE CANCER:

In cancer treatment, no word is more controversial than the word "cure." This is so because in the first place it is difficult to cure cancer, and in the second it is difficult to know when it has been cured. Even when doctors are reasonably sure that a cure has been accomplished, the nature of the disease makes it difficult to confirm this with the certainty with which one can proclaim, for instance, that a case of bronchitis has been cured. With cancer—a varied, capricious, tenacious disease— it's not quite so simple.

Part of the problem is that cancers grow at different rates. Their progress is unpredictable. They may grow back slowly or astoundingly quickly after a seemingly successful course of treatment has been completed. Take, for example, the frequently heard term "five-year survival," which is often equated with a cure. Some patients believe once they have passed the five-year mark, they are cured once and for all. Others are under the impression that even though they have been disease-free all that time their disease will reoccur after five years are up. Others aren't quite sure what it means.

In actuality, once some cancer patients pass this benchmark and are without symptoms they can breathe more easily because the chances for a recurrence are sharply diminished. However, while this is true for *some* cancers, it is by no means true for *all*. With some, it takes less time to start talking about a cure.

In the case of some cancers, such as leukemia, Burkitt's lymphoma, and testicular cancer, two years is enough time to pronounce a cure. With others, such as breast, thyroid, or bladder cancer, and with melanoma, eight to ten or more years must pass before we can begin to entertain thoughts of a cure. However, even with these stubborn types, the chance of a recurrence decreases with each passing year. Statistically, patients who survive for five years after diagnosis have, on the average, an 85 percent chance of surviving for twenty years. Five-year survival rates, then, have some meaning for some cancers and are useful when talking in terms of general averages. It is not an arbitrary cutoff date, but neither is it some universal magic number.

Compounding the growth-rate problem is the newness of much of the treatment. How do you know if someone is cured if the therapy is only five years old? If even a single cancer cell escapes treatment, it may reproduce and form a recurrence somewhere—perhaps twenty years down the line. Modern, organized, scientifically controlled chemotherapy is barely fifteen years old; some forms are only a few years old when they reach patients, and there are always the even newer experimental therapies.

Therefore, doctors would much rather stick to terms such as "no evidence of disease" (NED) and "remission." NED or full remission means that the patient has no cancer that is detectable using the techniques that are presently available. Since a person can be alive after five (or ten) years and still have (undetected or detected) cancer, these are much more cautious, though more accurate and realistic, terms that are usually used for several years after treatment.

In *Cancer Facts and Figures 1983*, the American Cancer Society lists the following cancers that a few decades ago had poor prognoses and that today are being cured in many cases, even though the disease may be widespread, primarily because of chemotherapy advances: acute lymphocytic leukemia, adult myelogenous leukemia, Hodgkin's disease, diffuse histiocytic lymphoma, Burkitt's lymphoma, nodular mixed lymphoma, Ewing's sarcoma, Wilms's tumor, rhabdomyosarcoma, choriocarcinoma, testicular cancer, ovarian cancer, breast cancer, and osteogenic sarcoma. Many people are being cured due to the success of adjuvant chemotherapy, which will be discussed next.

Most chemotherapy given with an intent to cure widespread cancer is aggressive, high-dose, and highly toxic. The side effects can be severe and complications requiring hospitalization are more common. However, because the chances are so good for a cure, most people feel the risks are worth it. For them, the time lost to chemotherapy—usually a year or less—is a reasonable price to pay for the chance of living out a normal life-span.

TO PREVENT OR DELAY A RECURRENCE OR SPREAD (ADJUVANT CHEMOTHERAPY):

Chemotherapy is being given earlier and earlier in some types of cancers, before metastases are detectable. By administering the drugs soon after surgery or radiotherapy has eradicated the bulk of the tumor, the chances are high that the drugs will be able to mop up the microscopic stragglers left behind. The goal is to wipe out the small numbers of circulating cells before they have time to settle down and grow into secondary tumors. Thus, a recurrence is at least delayed; time may prove it to be prevented altogether and the patient cured.

The concept of adjuvant chemotherapy began to be tested only in the early 1970s. But since then evidence has been accumulating to show that it does work in several cancers—mostly children's cancers such as Wilms's tumor and osteogenic carcinoma. Many women have also responded to adjuvant chemotherapy for breast cancer, though researchers and clinicians say it is still too early to tell whether it is effective for this tenacious disease that many not recur for twenty years.

Adjuvant chemotherapy should be given only to people whose disease has been carefully diagnosed and who have a high risk of recurrence, and only when there are drugs available that have been proven effective against their type of cancer. This is the case with breast cancer when there are more than four positive lymph nodes—a woman has a 75 percent chance of a recurrence within ten years, even though a mastectomy removed all detectable traces of cancer—and in osteogenic sarcoma, which has an 80 percent chance of recurring with lung metastases within a year after surgery. However, the encouraging results of adjuvant chemo studies with these cancers suggest other cancers may respond as well because it is now suspected that microscopic colonies of cancer cells are present in the majority of cancer patients with solid tumors.

As a result, adjuvant chemo is being given for other cancers, but the practice is controversial because it may prove to be more harmful than beneficial: In some cancers patients have actually done worse, and the cancer recurs earlier and with greater frequency than in patients who have not had the drugs. (No one knows why, but perhaps it is because the drugs weaken the body too much.)

The decision to undergo adjuvant chemotherapy is in some ways harder to make than that for other types of chemo. The chances are overwhelming that the micrometastases are there, but there's always a chance that there is no spread or that the body will be able to control the remaining cancer cells naturally. This is chemotherapy as an insurance policy and it is difficult to justify at the time because there's no concrete proof, except for past experience and statistical probability, that cancer is still there. The patient feels well; there is no discernible disease; and he or she may undergo all those side effects for nothing. Dr. Van Scoy-Mosher's concern that his patients understand adjuvant chemotherapy led him to write a booklet for his breast cancer patients who receive this type of therapy. He is aware that it presents quite unique and troublesome issues:

> "I find adjuvant chemotherapy for breast cancer is one of the most interesting and challenging things in the world to give. Because the questions that come up all the time are: How do you know it's needed? How do you know it's working? The only news in adjuvant chemotherapy is bad news. As long as I find nothing, that's good news.
>
> "I make it clear to patients that I don't know if they need it—there's no way of knowing because the surgery might have cured them to start with. And as years go by and the patient remains fine, I'll never know whether that's because of the therapy or whether she would have been fine anyway. And if that bothers me, I can imagine how it would make the patient crazy: The therapy's a drag, you get sick, maybe you didn't need it. At some level, you're going to have to take this on faith: that my educated guess is the right one."

Lari Wenzel, former director of the Cancer Information Service at the Comprehensive Cancer Center for the State of Florida, thinks:

"People who undergo this type of therapy have a great will to live. They also have some advantages. They know that they will not be on these drugs forever: It is not an infinite process. They know that their disease is fairly local or in an early stage. I think it really helps to tackle something like chemotherapy knowing that your chances of getting well are so great. The decision to choose chemotherapy is much different for people with advanced disease. They must hope for disease control and palliation."

TO CONTROL CANCER:

Even when a cancer isn't cured, it may be controlled for a time by chemotherapy. The goals here are to stop or slow down the growth of a tumor, or shrink it at least partially (partial remission), and to alleviate any pain, bleeding, obstruction, or other symptoms of the cancer (palliation). As a result, some patients feel better and live longer.

Although, as we have seen, cancer can be a curable disease, the idea of controlling cancer so people can still live with it reflects one current medical view of cancer as a chronic disease. By definition, a chronic disease is not curable; on the other hand, it is treatable, and people don't usually die from it right away. Dr. Charles Vogel of the University of Miami's Comprehensive Cancer Center explains:

"When one speaks about incurable cancer, as in the case of some metastatic disease, that's a chronic disease. But even with people who have had a recurrence, though we usually can't cure them, we can maintain these people's normal life-styles, without hospitalization, for three, four, five, eight, or ten years. This isn't commonly realized even by my medical colleagues. There is a gestalt that equates cancer with imminent death. When we talk about chronic disease we talk about people with arthritis, congestive heart failure, emphysema, multiple sclerosis. You can't cure these, but you can give people drugs and keep them functioning. Many types of cancer fit into that category."

The cancers that are usually not curable but may be controlled by chemotherapy include: cancer of the mouth, esophagus, stomach, colon, rectum, pancreas, bladder, cervix, liver, skin, brain, lung (nonoat cell), and malignant melanomas. In addition, the cancers listed earlier are not always cured by the initial treatment, but they may be controlled for a time.

When chemotherapy for palliation is offered, it is crucial to weigh the severity of the symptoms against the toxicity of the drugs and the expected response rate to the drug. Also considered are the patient's age and general health, the cost of treatment, and where it will be given. When cure is not a realistic hope, the minuses may outweigh the pluses. It may not be worthwhile to begin or continue treatment if a few extra months of life are spent feeling nauseated, vomiting, and being away from family and friends.

Cure, preventing or delaying recurrence, and palliation— these are the main goals of chemotherapy and it is important that you understand the difference. As Dr. Thomas Hakes, a physician at Memorial Sloan-Kettering in New York, says, "When you're trying to decide whether to go on chemotherapy or not, you should have a clear understanding of what you are trying to accomplish. People often have unrealistic expectations."

After asking your oncologist what the goal is in your case, you can also ask what the likelihood is of achieving that goal. The "response rate" varies from treatment to treatment; the average rate at which patients respond to a specific treatment is based on a statistical analysis of past experience, and this rate differs in different treatments. For example, the cure rate may be 50 percent or more, as in Hodgkin's disease or metastatic testicular cancer; or there may be a 15 percent chance of temporary improvement, as with metastatic melanoma. Awareness of such response rates can be useful when deciding upon a treatment.

But beware of the doctor who tells you how long you have to live; even though the doctor may be correct statistically, patients and their cancers are highly individual. Statistics are based on average figures for a group of patients with the same type and stage of cancer who get the same treatment. To get this average number, patients who lived much shorter periods of time and those who lived much longer were included. While statistical comparisons are valuable for comparing overall results of treatments, no one can ever say with certainty at which end of the spectrum any one particular patient will fall. Dr. Philip Schulman, an oncologist at North Shore University Hospital in New York, feels that "percentages simply don't mean anything. Each individual is either 100 percent or zero percent. Nobody wants to gamble with his or her life, and that's what percentages are."

OTHER FACTORS

Whether you're a gambler or not, percentages are not the only issue. Dr. Van Scoy-Mosher enumerates some of the many other factors that influence patients' decisions to have chemotherapy or not:

"You have to consider the cancer and the stage, the symptoms or problems with cancer they are having, what kind of longevity they are likely to have, the question of them getting much sicker from the cancer—these are medical issues.

"There's a real dilemma in evaluating the cost-benefit ratio: What's the realistic goal of this therapy—what am I likely to do *for* the patient as opposed to what am I likely to do *to* the patient? How do you balance those two things? Is a little longer life, but a sicker one, worth it? Or is just the chance of a longer life worth the certainty of a lot of side effects?

"Then there is a whole set of issues related to the individual person—age, psychology, expectations, family structure, which is something very important—some are under a lot of pressure from their family to take chemo. You have to blend all these.

"It's a complex decision to make in some patients; other situations are fairly clear-cut to me. If a person has advanced Hodgkin's disease, I know realistically I can probably cure him with chemicals. Assuming he wants to live, I don't see a big dilemma there. If there's a person with breast cancer with positive nodes, I am quite convinced that chemotherapy is a good idea and will recommend it very strongly. Then there are the marginal situations where chemotherapy may or may not help for a short period of time. Here's when you have to consider the other factors. Then there are other situations where I think chemotherapy is far more likely to make someone worse than better. The decision not to give chemotherapy is easy in those patients. What's harder is telling them."

Chemotherapy, for instance, is not for anyone whose diagnosis has not been confirmed via biopsy, whose tumor has not been staged and graded via X rays, scans, and other diagnostic tests. In addition, chemo may be too much of a strain on you physically and mentally if your general health is weak. Poor nutritional status or digestion, liver or kidney problems, infection, and other conditions may preclude, postpone, or modify the treatment with chemotherapy.

Dr. Gralla thinks this is a "very important point." He says:

"Chemotherapy works best in people who are not greatly disabled by the cancer. There's a certain point beyond which I don't believe chemotherapy is a good choice for a patient. If there's a chance that it will do more harm than good, I try to talk with the patients and their families and explain the situation. If they insist—'I really want the treatment'—I can say 'We can try to get you up to the point where you're strong enough for chemo—use antibiotics, nutrition, pain medicine. Then maybe yes. But I'm not comfortable giving you this, I don't think it's a good idea.'

"Sometimes I'm criticized by my colleagues outside this hospital because in general I will not treat people's lung cancer with drugs unless they are capable of being an outpatient. If somebody's bedridden then they're usually too sick for drug therapy for lung cancer. This is not the case with some other cancers such as leukemia or lymphoma. But you have to know the patient and find out what his or her philosophy is. Everybody's different, both in terms of outlook and physical condition at the time of presentation."

To help you make this all-important decision, you can refer to any one or several comprehensive books on cancer care. These include Harold Glucksberg and Jack W. Singer, *Cancer Care*; Charles F. McKhann, *The Facts About Cancer*; Kathryn H. Salsbury and Eleanor L. Johnson, *The Indispensable Cancer Handbook*; and Marion Morra and Eve Potts, *Choices*. They contain individual chapters on specific cancers and their treatments and are excellent sources of information about the many aspects of cancer. (These and other books are listed in the Bibliography.) *The Indispensable Cancer Handbook* suggests that you also go to a medical library and read articles about your cancer that have been published in professional journals within the last three years. These may be difficult for the average person to understand, but they will provide the names of doctors and institutions that specialize in your type of cancer and that you can contact for advice.

Ideally, the therapy and its ramifications should be discussed with one or more people who are close to you and who will be involved in your life while you undergo the treatment. They are the ones who can help support you during treatment if and when you need it. Together with a few health professionals whose judgment you trust—nurses, social workers, your family doctor—they can form a network of helpers who can offer to gather facts about alternate therapies, including alternate chemo protocols, support services, side effects, and economics. They can also help sort out conflicting information, evaluate and "translate" technical information, and participate in your making decisions based on that information.

I decided to have chemo because it seemed to be my best chance to continue to live and be well, to be cured. Even though I knew there would be side effects, and that chemo was no guarantee, it was still the lesser of two evils. People decide to have chemo because they believe it will give them something they need and want. What it gives in return might be a cure, it might be a few extra years of life, it might only be hope which makes life bearable. Whatever the reason, it is a positive choice, a vote for life, which seems more precious because it is being threatened, and a vow to fight to the best of your ability to enjoy your life for as long as you can.

Many people are alive today because they decided the risk of chemotherapy was worth taking. Many others have lived beyond expectation, long enough to accomplish important goals such as completing the writing of a book, seeing a daughter graduate from college, enjoying the birth of a grandson. Even those who were not cured were able to share a few more precious moments with people close to them, to buy extra time to come to grips with their illness, take care of business, say goodbye.

Barbara Blumberg, a public health educator with the National Cancer Institute's Cancer Information Service, sums up her attitude this way:

"In the past few years there have been a lot of different things done to help patients get through the drugs, from new antiemetic [antinausea] drugs to people recognizing that some of the nonmedical methods to help people relax are really useful.

"We know so little, but we do know there are a lot of treatments that do a lot of good for a lot of people with cancer. If I had cancer and could have chemotherapy, those are the statistics I would go by. I know I'm a person, not a statistic, but look at all the people who have done well."

IS STANDARD OR INVESTIGATIONAL CHEMOTHERAPY FOR YOU?

STANDARD CHEMOTHERAPY

It has been estimated by the National Cancer Institute and others that 250,000 to 400,000 people receive chemotherapy each year. Most of them receive the standard therapy for their particular form of cancer: The drug or combination of drugs that has been proven to be the best treatment available "off the shelf." All drugs used in standard treatment have been tested to the satisfaction of the Food and Drug Administration and approved for use. The medical profession is confident that it knows enough about the side effects so that these drugs pose an acceptable amount of risk in relation to the benefits they offer. No formal consent form needs to be signed for standard therapy; the physician simply tells the patient what the known possible risks and benefits are, and if the patient accepts the treatment, treatment is begun soon afterward.

However, standard therapy does not work for every cancer patient or it may have only minimal effect: in some cancers, no effective standard therapy exists. These patients are usually offered new experimental chemotherapy that may be more effective.

EXPERIMENTAL OR
INVESTIGATIONAL CHEMOTHERAPY

Approximately 36,000 or 18 percent of patients who accept chemotherapy receive experimental, or investigational, treatments. These experiments, in effect, put new, promising treatments on trial. If one proves itself to be more effective than any standard treatment, it too becomes standard. And if a treatment is at least equal to other established treatments but is toxic in a different way, it becomes an alternate standard therapy useful for some patients.

In chemotherapy, studies are needed to test each new drug individually, to test drugs in new combinations, to test using standard drugs in new ways, and to directly compare two types of treatments, each of which is known to be effective. The development and widespread use of a new drug is a long, complex, expensive process involving testing cancer in test tubes, laboratory animals, and humans. Human testing itself goes through three phases. It takes an average of eight to twelve years for a drug to progress from discovery to acceptance, and it costs millions of dollars. (This process is explained on pp. 290–94.)

Since less is known about the new drugs being tested than about the old standard drugs, it is difficult, if not impossible to come up with a realistic cost-benefit ratio. Because of this, some people derisively call those who participate in trials "guinea pigs." In some small sense, they are. But real guinea pigs are not asked to sign consent forms; they are not given any options in their treatments. But people are. It is true that human subjects are taking a gamble, but it should be their informed decisions to do so. Participating in an investigational trial gives patients an opportunity to receive state-of-the-art treatment—warts and all—that would not otherwise be available, and that can make a vast difference in their prognoses. Though these studies can vary tremendously in their risk to the patient, there is always an implied double benefit: Both the patient and the discipline of medical oncology can gain. In addition, some feel that a patient gets better all-round treatment in a clinical trial because there are strict criteria for control. The diagnosis must be specific and confirmed, the staging complete, and the required laboratory tests done. Patients are thoroughly monitored during and after treatment. This is true even if a patient is randomized—assigned by chance—to a standard therapy.

As a result of investigational chemotherapy, some people are helped, some are cured, but many are not. Some get sicker because of the drugs, some even die because of them. (However, patient deaths are still more frequently caused by the cancer than by the investigational drug.)

Experimental chemotherapy is given by "investigators"—physicians who are usually highly trained and qualified to specialize in cancer care, and who conduct studies. They must have access to laboratory and hospital support facilities. If the therapy is very new and highly experimental, it may be given only at comprehensive cancer centers or university hospitals. Recently more and more investigational therapies are becoming available from physicians at community hospitals or from physicians in private practice. These usually would not normally have enough patients of their own to complete a study. To overcome this deficit, cooperative oncology groups have been established. Doctors who are members participate in cooperative studies that include patients in other cities with similar cancers. Recently, CCOP, a new program, has been instituted to involve more local physicians. Cooperative group studies and their affiliated CCOP-member studies help ensure that enough patients will be found to complete the study and to make experimental treatment available to a larger segment of the population. Your local physician can make arrangements for you to be included in a study. In some cases, patients undergoing investigational therapies are treated without charge. Not everyone who applies will be accepted—you must fit the needs of the group.

Anyone who enters an investigational study must sign an "informed consent" form. These vary from institution to institution and from group to group, but in general the form tells the patient the known possible side effects and the possible benefits to be expected from the treatment.

Informed consent forms are written by the institution or group conducting the study. To ensure adequacy and accuracy, each form is reviewed and approved by the institution's own Institutional Review Board (IRB) and then by the NCI. Thus, many experts have examined it before the patient is asked to sign and the study can proceed.

If you are contemplating investigational therapy, the informed consent form should be only a jumping off point for healthy discussions between you and your doctor. Study it carefully. It may not contain all the information you need to make your decision. If you want to know more, ask your doctor. He or she should be willing to explain the treatment thoroughly and honestly tell you what benefits you might derive. In all cases, be sure there is no alternate therapy that you might prefer. In very recently developed treatments especially, ask about what is already known about the drug—whether it has worked for other cancer patients and what the rare side effects might be. Find out how many people with your type of cancer have received the therapy and how many have responded. Knowing that others were helped by this treatment might influence your decision, no matter what the risks. Remember, you have the right to refuse this treatment, or to discontinue it at any time.

You might want to consider experimental therapy simply because it's better than doing nothing. If you are the type of person who refuses to give up, who will try anything to live longer, investigational therapy may provide you with more than a physical therapy—it can help you psychologically. Some patients' motivation is the emotional satisfaction they derive from knowing that they are helping others who might benefit from the therapy in the future.

Dr. Thomas Hakes explains:

"A person who gets an investigational drug is someone for whom we have exhausted all standard therapy. At this point we can only treat the patients symptomatically, to try and make them comfortable and allow them to go about their business as best they can. Or we can try investigational drugs, which we certainly cannot guarantee are going to help. By their very nature they're not likely to help because we go through ten or fifteen investigational drugs for every one that turns out to be useful. A lot of people don't want them, but a surprising number of people do."

In general, the further along the investigation is, the higher the likelihood that you will benefit. In phase I, the chances are small. Usually very little is known about the drug. Therapeutic effect may be seen in phase I, but since doses may be below the ideal therapeutic range, positive results often do not occur even in drugs that later prove to be effective. An estimated 10 percent of patients respond to phase I drugs.

A doctor who offers a patient a phase I investigational drug is saying in effect: "We know of nothing that will help you. But we have a new drug that might. It might also make you worse, and you might die sooner than you would without it. But if you take it, I will be watching you very carefully to try to prevent anything really bad from happening." Some of these adverse reactions may not be predictable from the animal studies—mice, rats, dogs, and apes do not react exactly like human beings. These preclinical studies usually do reveal liver and kidney toxicity, but they may not alert investigators to possible damage to the central nervous system, heart, lungs, and skin in humans.

Toward the end of a phase I trial, some encouraging data might have come in about the drug, and you might be able to find out if the drug has helped anyone else, particularly with your type of cancer. In addition, more will be known about the range of therapeutic dosage. This bit of knowledge can significantly shift the odds in your favor.

Since there is no accepted form of effective treatment for people who are offered phase I drugs, some may prefer to have no therapeutic treatment. The may prefer to let the disease run its course without the additional discomfort that chemotherapy can bring.

It is a bold, brave soul who accepts phase I treatment. In their book *Cancer Care,* Drs. Harold Glucksberg and Jack W. Singer write:

> "We urge that you carefully consider whether you want to enter a phase I trial. We definitely do not feel it is worthwhile for you to travel to a medical center not in your community to receive a phase I drug. If the drug is available in your community, there are only two reasons for trying it: It offers hope and it may help others with cancer."

For phase II subjects, the outlook is better. At least most of the side effects and dose limitations are known. Still, it is usually uncertain whether the drug is effective in human cancers, let alone which types are most likely to respond. So the chances that you will benefit are still rather small. However, it is possible that someone with your type of cancer did respond to this drug. In the early stages of a phase II there may be

some positive data from phase I, and in the later stages of a
phase II there may be some good news from the previous studies
done in this phase. So ask your doctor—if you happen along
at the end of a phase II that has shown good responses to your
type of cancer, it could mean a dramatic difference in your
prognosis.

A doctor who offers a patient a phase II drug is saying: "We
have very little standard therapy that can help you. We think
we have a drug that might work in your type of cancer; we're
pretty sure it won't harm you severely, and we have a very
good idea of what to watch out for."

Phase III trials are usually the safest of all. By the time a
drug reaches this point, it has gone through enough testing so
that doctors know which cancers respond to it, how much they
respond, and what the side effects are. You are offered this
treatment only if it has already been proven that it is effective
in your type of cancer.

If you are offered phase III treatment, your doctor is saying:
"We have standard drugs that we know will help you. But we
think we have something that may be even better. The investigational arm of the study consists of a recipe (protocol) that
we have a tremendous amount of confidence is just as good as
the conventional arm, and that we think is better. This study
compares the two treatments and we think will prove that the
new is better." So with phase III the patient is not taking much
more of a gamble than if he or she took conventional therapy.

GETTING A SECOND OPINION

The rationale for getting a second opinion is getting stronger
every day. As cancer care has improved over the last decades,
it has gotten more complex and sophisticated. If you have any
lingering doubts about your diagnosis or the recommended
treatment, you should definitely consider getting a second, and
even perhaps a third, opinion by consulting with another expert
in the field. (Be sure to find out from your oncologist how
much time you have to decide—some cancers do not require
immediate treatment, but a delay in others could alter your
prognosis dramatically.) Being dissatisfied with the therapeutic
effects of your treatment, the side effects and the way they are
handled, or an irreconcilable doctor-patient personality conflict

are other possible motivating factors for getting a second opinion.

Training, capabilities, and philosophies vary greatly; no one can expect every doctor to have learned everything in his field, even if he is a specialist. Some stay more up-to-date than others by attending seminars and conventions and reading many journals; some have a more aggressive approach to disease than others. Some have sub-subspecialties, such as bone cancer, or breast cancer, or lung cancer. None of the conventional or investigational treatments is fun. You want to be sure to get the maximum return on whatever effects you suffer, and a consultation helps you do that.

Often a situation is not clear-cut, or new therapies are being developed. Dr. Thomas Hakes specializes in treating breast cancer at Memorial Sloan-Kettering and gives a lot of second opinions. "Often there are no real right answers or best answers," he says, "rather there are several possibilities." How often does he disagree with the first opinion? "I'd say 40 to 50 percent of the time I agree exactly; about 25 percent of the time it's not exactly what I would do, but it's still acceptable; and 25 percent of the time I disagree completely."

Going for a consult also gives you time to think, reflect, and digest—time that is invaluable for the coping process. Many health care professionals, including oncologists themselves, recognize the advantages of hearing someone else's views at any point during treatment. Consultations are especially important at the time of diagnosis, and many oncologists will routinely send biopsy slides to a second pathologist. You can ask whether this has been done—biopsies examined in small communities by a lone pathologist are prime candidates for second opinions at larger institutions such as cancer centers, major medical centers, or university medical centers. The finer points of a diagnosis can dictate crucial differences in your prognosis and treatment.

Though justifiable, asking for a second opinion is not always easy. Patricia Henry, an oncology nurse at New York's Memorial Sloan-Kettering, points out that "there's a certain gut feeling you have about a doctor. If you like him and trust him, you may be reluctant to see someone else. It's hard to break in a new doctor." For some patients, such as this one, the idea never occurs. "This whole thing was rather new to me—though I suppose it is to everybody. I never thought about my alternatives. I just trusted my doctors and did what they told me."

Other cancer patients, no matter how they long for a confirmation or consultation, are timid about suggesting it. "I don't want to hurt my doctor's feelings," they say, or "I'm afraid my doctor won't treat me if I go see someone else." This lung cancer patient, for example, was very unhappy with the treatment her oncologist, who was affiliated with a top cancer center, was giving her:

> "I was so violently ill—I thought dying couldn't be worse. So I went to the Cancer Management Center in Kansas City for another opinion. My doctor was very angry with me. But I said, 'Doctor, I *need* this.' Finally he agreed to forward my records. The panel at Kansas City told me the way I was being treated was *the way*, if I was to survive this. That put my mind at ease; it was the best five hundred dollars I ever spent."

Most oncologists, however, enourage their patients to tap another expert's thoughts. Dr. Michael Van Scoy-Mosher is one:

> "I might want to hear what another doctor has to say. Somewhere early on, I bring it up with the patients, just so they don't view it as an insult to my ego. I really like my patients to know that they can do that. The other thing I do is ask that they let me guide them a little bit about where to get that second opinion. I want to be sure it's from a reputable, well-respected oncologist. They also must understand that when you seek another opinion, you risk actually *getting* another opinion—and that you will then have to reconcile the conflict."

Though you may find a good oncologist locally, he may not have access to all the benefits of the explosion of knowledge in the cancer field. He should, however, make sure that somehow *you* do have access. Most smaller local hospitals do have tie-ins with nearby larger centers. The key is for you to be able to discuss the need for expert consultation with your doctor and have his willingness to cooperate.

If you do go for a second opinion, the names of consulting physicians may be obtained and their credentials and affiliations checked out by using the same channels and methods suggested for finding a first physician. In addition, your first physician may be more than happy to recommend other specialists.

In their book, *Choices: Realistic Alternatives in Cancer Treatment*, Marion Morra and Eve Potts suggest that if you are hesitant about broaching the subject with your doctor, enlist the aid of a relative or friend. They can supply moral support or courage when you explain your need to your physician or perhaps do the explaining for you. The authors point out that a concurring second opinion will strengthen your physician's conclusions and make you feel more secure, confident, and at ease with the treatment. Belief in the treatment seems to have a strong effect on how well a patient does with chemotherapy. If your doctor is offended at the suggestion of getting another opinion, Morra and Potts suggest that you get another doctor.

I remember when my oncologist outlined the course of the chemo he planned for me. The next week, when I came back to start the treatment, he told me he'd found that an older protocol for adjuvant breast cancer chemotherapy was more effective than the one currently in vogue. It called for slightly different drugs, a different schedule, and lasted nine months rather than the year the other therapy stipulated. I was glad about the relative brevity of the plan, but I also felt a vague uneasiness about the therapy. I wondered: Is there yet another therapy that's even more effective? In spite of this, I never went for a second opinion. It wasn't until I researched this book that I inadvertently got a belated "second opinion" from one of the oncologists I interviewed: He confirmed that my oncologist "knew what he was doing" and I breathed a huge sigh of relief. Three years is a long time to wait for that kind of reassurance, no matter how slight your doubt.

When calling for an appointment, make it clear that you are interested in a consultation; arrangements will have to be made for your records and test results to be forwarded. Although the consulting physician could end up treating you if you prefer, you are not obligated to stay with the last doctor you see.

Dr. Isadore Rosenfeld, in his book *Second Opinion: Your Medical Alternatives*, sums up the case for getting a second opinion:

> "No matter how devoted you are to your doctor or how much you dislike antagonizing him, you owe it to yourself to consult with another expert when you are ill and not responding to treatment, or when you are presented

witn a diagnosis, prognosis, or recommendation that may drastically alter the course of your life. . . .

"Your doctor usually has several alternatives at his disposal to treat most conditions. One may be better, more convenient, or more appropriate for you than another. You should know—or be made aware of—all these options when you are sick, and you should be able to discuss them freely with your physician. Unfortunately either because they are too busy, or don't believe that it's really any of your business, some doctors don't tell you that you have any choice at all, or what it is. That attitude is not in your best interest, nor is it likely to result in the best medical care for you."

Help For The Mind,
Body, And Spirit

CHAPTER 5

Coping With Chemotherapy

Whether you are still in the process of deciding on a therapy, about to begin treatment, or already on it, it is important to remember that many people before you have gone through chemo, that they did manage to cope, and that there are ways that have been developed to help you get through it too. The same strength that stems from the will to live and enables people to make the tough decision to undergo chemo continues to stand them in good stead during the actual treatment. So do a positive attitude, a good doctor-patient relationship, a strong and reliable support system, and a realistic picture of what to expect in the way of results and side effects.

Dr. Michael Van Scoy-Mosher, an oncologist at Cedars-Sinai Medical Center in Los Angeles, believes that "it's very important for most patients to have an understanding of what the therapy is all about, what its purpose is, what its goals are—and to have a certain attitude about it that the therapy is more an ally than an enemy. It is the disease that is the enemy."

Barbara Blumberg, a public health educator at the National Cancer Institute, thinks it's important for people to keep in mind the reason why they're doing the chemotherapy—that it's for the ultimate good. "You have to be goal-oriented because the way to that goal is not that wonderful."

Lari Wenzel, former director of the Cancer Information

Service at the Comprehensive Cancer Center for the State of Florida, says:

> "People who want to know as much as possible about their disease and treatment, why they are experiencing side effects and that these side effects can be controlled—those people tend to do well because their attitude and approach allow them an active role in fighting their disease. People should try to retain their life-styles as much as possible so that they are not identifying themselves only as cancer patients undergoing chemotherapy, but rather thinking that this is one event among many that is taking place in their lives. People who are able to work, even part-time—if they can retain their work identity and family identity—tend to cope better."

Patients have their own theories about coping too:

> "When you're so very sick, you go through all these emotions. You're angry and sorry for yourself at first. And then you say, 'Hey, I'm not going to let this get me down.' I just made up my mind I wasn't going to have to worry about who was going to raise my daughter. I was going to do it myself."

> "I guess everybody handles it in his or her own way. There's no set answer. If you're religious, you pray. If you're not, you turn to an inner strength. But behind all of us, there has to be some stirring, some push. Because we're all afraid. When you're told you're going to die, you'll put yourself through anything to be able to live."

> "It wasn't easy, but you learn. Friends would pitch in when my wife wasn't there to help me. We all worked together. Somehow, you just *do* it."

> "The mind has to really take over the body. If you let what they are doing to your body really sink in and go to your head—chances are you won't make it. I just stopped thinking about my body being systematically poisoned, the fact that I was agreeing to it, paying for it, and even putting some of it in my mouth myself."

With the admirable resilience, adaptability, and ingenuity that characterize the human race, most patients do manage to adjust to living in what has been called chemotherapy's "twilight world" of not being really sick, but not being really well either. In spite of the side effects, great and small, physical and emotional, most people find that they are able to live fairly normal, satisfying lives while on chemotherapy. They continue to work, play, eat, socialize, go to school, take care of their households and families, and even travel pretty much as usual, at least most of the time.

In most cases, chemotherapy is only a temporary way of life, but it is still a life that must be lived. Regardless of your prognosis, you can have a rich and rewarding life if you make every moment count. There is no reason to deprive yourself unnecessarily. Every avenue should be explored that will help you live fully within your real—and not your imagined—limitations. It may take some extra effort and planning by you and those who care about you; adjustments, and perhaps some substitutions may have to be made. You may need to set up new priorities. But there is usually some way to do the things that are most important to you. There *is* more to life than cancer and chemotherapy.

If you find you are particularly bothered or concerned about a side effect, refer to the individual chapters on side effects (Chapters 10–15) and the chapters on support services (Chapters 6–9). Be sure to report your side effects to your doctor, who should have some suggestions that may help. For example, it's quite common to have a few days after a treatment when you feel more or less out of commission, and you simply have to take it easy. No one should expect to maintain a full schedule of activities when saddled with nausea, vomiting, or just plain overwhelming weakness. Eventually, a certain rhythm will take hold; you may learn to dread this part of the cycle, or actually welcome, in some strange way, the quiet days. Should your life be too disrupted, nutritional support, household help, physical activity, or psychosocial counseling can often help to alleviate your troubles. Remember that schedules can be adjusted so your worst days coincide with the times you least mind having to take it easy, be it weekends or workdays, and most dosages and drugs can be adjusted too.

My ability to cope was certainly helped by a relatively good prognosis, a supportive husband-to-be, a compassionate, optimistic oncologist who added nutritional therapy and encouraged me to exercise, the ability to continue to work and keep my sense of humor, and the means to escape reality for a few moments by focusing on something other than chemotherapy.

We all learn to cope because we have to—the alternative is much worse. We choose chemotherapy because no matter what the price we pay—in time, money, side effects, and emotional energy—the benefits are greater than without it. Whether chemo gives us a cure, a few extra years, or only hope, our will to live is what gives us the wherewithal to find and utilize whatever inner and outer help is available. Outside support makes it easier and removes some of the strain; but nothing can make chemo go away completely. The stubborn daily reality—the dark side of chemo—always remains. And after a certain point that can only be ignored or denied.

Ultimately it is something within ourselves that allows us to make that extra effort to tough it out. Chemo for me seemed very much like life itself, only more so: a great challenge and a great adventure. I had my ups and downs, but I learned to take one day at a time. I tried to not expect the worst, not to think too much about the bad things that might happen—only the good ones.

GETTING INFORMATION

Being well informed is widely recognized as essential to the coping process. Most people fear the unknown more than anything; the fantasies they conjure up are often far worse than the real thing. A reasonable amount of information can put anxieties to rest or at least into perspective. Since your oncologist knows the most about your particular case—your disease and its treatment—he or she should ideally be your primary source of information. Yet what patients want to know and what their doctors think they want to know rarely coincide.

Dr. Michael Van Scoy-Mosher thinks as a general rule that doctors tend to underestimate their patients' needs for information and understanding of their disease and its treatment. He feels they don't supply patients with nearly enough information and hesitate to bring up touchy issues on their own.

It's up to the patient to ask if more information is wanted. Patients are often hesitant to pose additional questions once the initial explanation has been provided or as the therapy wears on. Patients have many reasons for this: They say they are still in shock from the diagnosis, or they don't know what questions to ask, or they forget to ask, or they feel too shy and intimidated, or they don't want to look like fools, or they don't want to "waste" time asking silly questions of a busy doctor. Faced with an authority figure who knows more about us than we know about him, who has the power to cure, to heal, to relieve us of our pain, or to make us feel sicker, we can feel as though we are children who should be "seen but not heard."

Patients should not feel guilty about taking up a lot of their doctor's time—that's what the doctors are there for. Taking up time *unnecessarily* is another matter, so it is best to come prepared. When you are asking questions, there are several procedures you can follow so your queries are more effective. You can educate yourself by reading up on your disease and its treatment (your doctor can refer you to specific volumes and periodicals, or your librarian can). You can contact local branches of national cancer organizations such as the American Cancer Society and the National Cancer Institute's Cancer Information Service. They will give you information over the phone and send you booklets and articles pertinent to your disease. It is difficult to retain huge amounts of new information; at a time when your mind is under a lot of pressure, it is impossible. You can overcome this problem during visits to your doctor by bringing a pad and pencil and jotting down notes; or you can bring along a small cassette recorder and tape the whole conversation. Bringing a friend or family member with you is another possibility. They can remember things you don't, act as your health advocate by thinking up questions that you might not have, and pose questions you may not have the nerve to ask.

Many professionals suggest that you write down your questions as you think of them during the visit or during the time between visits. I didn't start writing down questions until well into the therapy for fear of feeling foolish. Finally, I decided it was more foolish not to. When I whipped out my list, my doctor just said, "Oh, a shopping list," and didn't bat an eyelash.

YOUR CHEMOTHERAPY PLAN

The chemotherapy plan (also referred to as a protocol, program, or regimen) is like a cooking recipe that specifies the drugs, the baseline doses of the drugs, and the scheduling of the treatments. Cancers as well as people vary in their responses to different plans, so in choosing a protocol, the oncologist tries to match your disease and general condition with the possible effectiveness and side effects of the thousands of available protocols. The plan he or she chooses and how it is implemented play a crucial role in how well you cope.

As you have seen, your chemotherapy may be standard or investigational; in addition, it may be a single drug (single agent chemotherapy), or your cancer might respond best to a multitude of drugs given simultaneously or sequentially (combination chemotherapy). You may be getting high-dose chemo, which is generally reserved for systemic cancers such as leukemias or lymphoma or for metastatic disease that has a good chance for a cure or remission. Or the chemo may be low-dose, which is used for adjuvant chemo and for palliation. The actual dose you get is usually calculated according to a formula based upon body weight or on total body surface area. Using the body surface area is more reliable because it tends to fluctuate less than body weight.

HOW MUCH LEEWAY?

Every effort is made to adhere to the established program as closely as is feasible because past experience shows that the treatment works best that way. An investigational protocol must be followed to the letter because it is a test, or else the results of the trial will be inaccurate. (However, a patient may be taken off a study and still receive some type of chemotherapy.)

But chemotherapy is not an all-or-nothing proposition. The goal in chemotherapy is to administer the "maximum tolerated dosage." This is the delicately balanced point at which as many cancer cells as possible are being killed without sacrificing too many normal cells. Too little of the drug, and too few cancer cells are killed; too much of it and too many normal cells are killed. When too many normal cells are affected, the therapy becomes too toxic and side effects become intolerable and possibly dangerous.

Everyone comes to chemotherapy with a different set of physical characteristics, and everyone reacts in a unique way. The art and science of giving chemotherapy well in part consists of knowing when and how to change a protocol so the patient is getting the best care. An oncologist will make changes in your treatment if the side effects are too debilitating or the drugs are not working well. Initially, a set protocol may be used intact, or drugs may be dropped and/or added. For instance, certain drugs may be toxic for a patient when a key organ is weak or malfunctioning. The anticancer drugs are processed and excreted by the liver and kidneys, so those organs are particularly stressed. But problems with other organs may mean that your doctor will have to give you less of a drug than it is standard to give, drop it from the plan entirely, or simply keep a very close watch on organs that he or she suspects may be dangerously affected.

Chemotherapy is commonly begun within a month after diagnosis since it is in part a race against time. Thereafter, the treatments are paced carefully. They must be given intermittently, in cycles, with enough time between treatments so that normal cells can reproduce and replace their lost sister cells in sufficient numbers to maintain an acceptable level of functions. However, there must not be so much time between treatments that the cancer cells can greatly recoup their losses.

Consequently, patients should try to make their treatments as scheduled, if possible on the exact day stipulated by their protocol, and to continue it for as long as the oncologist recommends. As with the drugs themselves, the timing and length of the therapy may be fine-tuned according to your response, your side effects, the goals of the treatment, and the availability of alternate treatments.

Chemotherapy protocols given with an intent to cure or bring about complete remission usually have a predetermined end date. These can last three months, six months, nine months, one year, two years, or three years. Experience has shown that on the average this is the least amount of time required to get the sought-after results, with acceptable side effects, in the greatest number of people.

Where the goal is partial remission, or when the protocol is investigational, the therapy is more open-ended. Chemotherapy may be relatively brief, a long constant haul, or an on-again, off-again proposition for the remainder of the patient's life. Drugs, doses, and schedules may be switched regularly in an attempt to prolong comfortable, productive life.

In cases of discernible disease, chemotherapy is given for as long as the drugs can be seen to be affecting the tumor and the patient is not suffering from severe side effects. The way the patient feels and various tests tell the doctor how well the drugs are working: Is the tumor still growing; if so, how fast? Has it stopped growing? Is it shrinking? It is gone?

If your tumor continues to grow or "progress" most oncologists will take you off chemotherapy or switch to a different group of drugs, no matter how well you tolerate the first group. They feel that if it continues to grow, despite various different drugs or combinations of them, chemotherapy is probably doing more harm than good; you are probably wasting your time, energy, and whatever health you have left. In some cases, a tumor whose growth has slowed down is an acceptable response and may continue to be treated with chemotherapy, provided that the side effects are tolerable. In others, a stable tumor (one that has stopped growing, but is not shrinking) may be the criterion for continuing.

If the tumor responds so well it actually shrinks (partial remission) chemotherapy may be continued until the tumor either no longer responds (i.e. shrinks) or begins to grow again; at this point other drugs are given, if possible, to which the tumor is not resistant. If the patient is in full remission with no detectable disease, chemotherapy may be continued on a maintenance basis, or stopped—it depends upon the cancer. Long-term remission can indicate a cure, but many remissions do not last forever; when the disease recurs, chemotherapy may be started up again with the same or new drugs.

Doctors use only very rough guidelines as to how much time the drugs should be given to work. As Dr. Richard Gralla, a doctor at New York's Memorial Sloan-Kettering, points out, it may depend upon many factors:

"For the most part, at least in the disease that I treat, which is lung cancer, you usually can tell within six to ten weeks whether a treatment is working. For instance, our first-line combination consists of a simple, easy medicine given weekly for a month and then every two weeks, and a difficult one given once a month. We usually wait until after the second difficult one—we like not to give the third injection unless we know that, yes, things are getting better.

"In breast cancer, though, it may be several months before you know whether hormone therapy is definitely helping. With most chemotherapy drugs—be they standard or investigational—the general range is four to ten weeks. With some people it's very easy to see if their tumors are getting bigger or smaller and if they're feeling better or not feeling better. For others it's not so easy to tell because you can't measure the disease very well and their symptoms may be complicated."

How much leeway to take in a chemotherapy regimen is one of the greatest dilemmas facing the oncologist—and one a cancer patient faces too, if he or she is an informed partner in the decisions concerning the treatment. Doctors often treat patients who are vomiting, who feel sick, whose blood counts are slipping, who are on the edge of developing any number of possibly serious additional ailments. How much toxicity is too much? At what point do you reduce, postpone, alter, or stop treatment even though you know it probably lessens the chance for a cure or a remission? A heart-to-heart discussion with your doctor should enable both of you to plan the right treatment program. Together you must take personal factors into consideration such as whether you need to keep on working or keep your household together.

In these cases, it is not advisable for your doctor to prescribe drugs that would knock you off your feet. You have to balance your emotional need to stay alert, capable, and "up" with the physical need to take strong chemotherapy to treat your cancer. There usually are a few choices to make.

If you suffer from immediate debilitating side effects and you need to stay well and alert because you are continuing to work, you can often schedule your appointments for late on a weekday or for a Friday. If weekends are important to you, you can have your treatments early in the week. Both these strategies will usually allow time for the worst of the immediate side effects to wear off in time for you to live your life pretty

much as planned. Because work was important to me, I got
my treatments on Friday: That way I could moan and mope
over the weekend, when the side effects were the worst. By
Monday I'd be ready to face the world again.

Itinerant chemotherapy patients can stay on schedule too,
with a little ingenuity. When I took a trip related to my work,
I didn't miss a shot (much as I would have liked to). I told my
oncologist my itinerary and he located a lab in one city, an
oncologist in another, and gave me my drugs to tote along. I
had two blood tests and one treatment away from home under
his long-distance guidance. Two weeks later I got off the plane
and had my next treatment, right on schedule.

THE METHODS

Chemotherapeutic drugs may be given in any of several
different ways, depending upon the dose, the preferences of
the doctor and the patient, and the type of cancer. The drugs
may be introduced into the body:

Orally (PO)—pills, capsules, or liquids taken by mouth
Intravenously (IV)—injected into a vein, either fast (IV
    push) or slow (IV drip or infusion)
Intramuscularly (IM)—Injected into a muscle
Subcutaneously (SQ)—injected underneath the skin
Intra-arterially (IA)—injected into an artery
Intrathecally (IT)—injected into the spinal fluid
Intracavitarily (IC)—injected into the pleural cavity of
    the chest or into the abdomen
Topically—applied directly to the skin, in the mouth or
    into the vagina

Most chemotherapy is given either orally or intravenously;
many protocols combine both methods. When given orally it
enters your bloodstream via the digestive system; intravenous
medication enters the blood directly via a vein. Once in the
bloodstream, the drug diffuses throughout the body and goes
to every cell of every organ supplied with blood by the cap-
illaries. The other methods are generally reserved for special
conditions to increase the drugs' effectiveness, reduce the side
effects, or both. For instance, a great deal of effort has been

made to give drugs intra-arterially, by *regional perfusion*. This method allows spot treatment of tumors whereby very high concentrations of drugs circulate only in the region of the tumor. Used in cases such as arm or leg tumors or liver metastases, the results of this method compare favorably with those of intravenous administration, with fewer side effects to the rest of the body. Intrathecal injections directly into the spinal fluid are another example. These are an attempt to overcome the blood-brain barrier and are often used in cancers such as leukemia that tend to spread to the central nervous system.

ORAL CHEMOTHERAPY

Some cancers are treated solely with oral chemotherapy. In many other protocols, oral drugs are used in addition to the injections. Your plan may call for you to take oral medication a few days every month, or everyday throughout the therapy. Since the pills, capsules, or liquid can be taken over the course of the day, oral administration allows a steadier supply of the drug to be circulating in the body.

Oral chemotherapy is particularly useful for patients who have "bad veins" and for whom IV chemotherapy is difficult, very painful, or impossible. However, it leaves the accuracy of the dosing up to the patient, and the pills themselves can have a horrible taste that stubbornly refused to be disguised. One patient comments:

"I took six pills a day, and they tasted so bitter. I can still taste them now, five years later. My oncologist suggested putting them in applesauce, but I don't like applesauce. I tried jelly, but that didn't work. I knew that people wrap pills for animals in chopped meat or bread, so I tried that for me, but they stuck in my throat. I'll never forget the taste."

Following the simple procedures will make pill taking easier. It is better to stand rather than to sit. Take a sip of water or other liquid to lubricate the throat to prevent the tablet from getting stuck. Then take a sip of liquid along with the pill and tilt the head back to swallow. Wash the pill down with a hefty chaser. It is important to remember to lubricate the throat first.

In the October 1982 issue of the *Journal of Nuclear Medicine*, a study by R. S. Fisher used X rays to reveal that medications stick in dry throats despite up to forty swallows and additional gulps of water.

If you are taking oral medication, it helps to establish a schedule that has some relation to your other activities. For instance, coordinate your pill taking with certain meals, or a favorite TV or radio show. Or a family member or neighbor may be able to remind you. Ask your doctor, nurse, or pharmacist to help you set up a workable schedule. Some drugs are best taken on an empty stomach, others on a full one. Some should not be taken just before bedtime. If you are taking a number of drugs by mouth, take care not to mix them up and to take each one at the proper time. If you are following a very complicated schedule, it may help to set out your medication for one day in a special container, or to keep a written record of your tablets. Another aid is to hang a large calendar near the location of your pills and mark large X's on the dates you are to take your pills. If you are taking several pills, use a different color pen to mark each medication.

If you miss a dose, check with your doctor about how to proceed. Sometimes you should take a missed dosage as soon as possible; sometimes you should not take the missed dose, or double up on the next dose to make it up, but rather continue as usual with the next scheduled dose.

Even though you may experience side effects from oral chemotherapy, you should not stop taking it or reduce the dosage on your own. Check with your doctor. He may prescribe different drugs, reduce the dose of your present drugs, prescribe additional drugs, or make suggestions that will alleviate the side effects.

Chemotherapy pills are very strong medications. As with all drugs, keep your chemotherapy pills out of the reach of children, and do not transfer them to anotehr drug container that might cause confusion and accidental dosing.

INTRAVENOUS CHEMOTHERAPY

For many drugs, IV injections are the preferred—or only—way for the drugs to enter your body. Drugs are usually given by IV because they reach more parts of the body that way, or because they are easier or cheaper to manufacture in that form.

Some drugs are absorbed only when they are given by injection. Some may be too irritating or unstable to be used in oral form.

Chemotherapy is most often injected into veins in the lower arm or hand because they are usually most accessible and convenient. Sometimes veins in other areas of the body are called upon when these are not usable.

There are two methods of giving an intravenous injection of chemotherapy drugs: push, and drip or infusion. The push is the fastest and simplest, but the method used for specific drugs on specific people depends upon which works best and which is least painful. Drugs given by the drip method are usually those that are deactivated very quickly; to increase the number of cells killed the drip method is used to maintain a certain level of the drugs for a long time. Sometimes a drug must be given slowly, in a diluted form, because it hurts the patient or results in adverse effects when it is given quickly.

An IV push takes five to fifteen minutes, depending upon the number of drugs, the size of the needle, and the ease with which the needle can be inserted into the vein. If you are getting combination chemotherapy, the doctor or nurse will insert a single needle into a vein and one by one feed a succession of drugs through the same needle to spare the vein from repeated piercings.

An IV drip takes longer—up to twelve hours for a single drug. For this technique, a needle is inserted into a vein and a bottle of the drug hangs from a pole. A thin tube connects the bottle to the needle and allows the drug to drip slowly at a steady rate into the vein. Some IV drip chemotherapy can be given on an outpatient basis. Patients who are on a protocol involving several drugs given by slow IV drip stay in the hospital for several days, and the IV needle remains in the vein for the duration of the treatment, with each drug administered in succession.

The sensations felt during the actual chemotherapy injection depend upon the skill of the oncologist or oncology nurse who administers the injection, the nature of the drugs, and the size and condition of the vein. A psychological component enters into it too—in some people fear and apprehension can make an unpleasant sensation feel worse.

Knowing this, I tried to relax as much as possible when the moment came. Eventually the treatments became less painful, less shocking, almost routine and normal. My oncologist had a skillful, gentle technique and used a tiny needle; still, a needle is a needle and I never got used to it completely. I looked away when he made the injection, especially when he was having trouble. Even though the pain was minimal compared to the surgery I'd been through, I couldn't stop a few tears from forming just the same—at that moment I'd feel sorry for myself all over again and I'd think, "Isn't it bad enough? I don't *need* this."

Some fortunate patients are endowed with huge, ropy veins, close to the surface of the skin. They never realize how lucky they are until chemotherapy enters their lives—"God may have given me cancer, but at least he gave me good veins." At the other end of the spectrum are the unfortunate ones with truly "bad veins"—small, thin-walled or tough-walled, or buried below the surface.

A good oncology nurse or doctor will do everything possible to make a vein more accessible to treatment and spare the patient discomfort. They may use ultrasmall needles and look for veins in odd places. Some try wrapping the arm with warm towels, or running warm water over the area to get the veins to come closer to the surface. Einstein Hospital's Dr. Ronald Bash recommends that his patients exercise, since this pumps up the veins: "It makes a modest difference but that's often enough. This is especially so in women undergoing chemotherapy for breast cancer, and who are getting injections in only one arm." My oncologist specifically recommended that I squeeze a rubber ball as often as possible to "pump up" the veins, but any exercise helps.

The drugs themselves—and the imagination and sensitivities of the patient—also impart unique sensations at injection time. A lot of the sensations are minor, localized, and temporary. Some patients say they feel a burning at the injection site; others feel a coldness or a warmth that spreads throughout the body and lasts for several minutes or more. Others feel an overall tingling, a chill, or a kind of "high." Some say they can "taste" their drugs within a few seconds of the beginning of the injection. I'd joke around and say, "Mmm—strawberry," and name another flavor every time. For other patients, the taste is no joke. For example: "That metallic taste would hit my mouth shortly after the infusion began. If I live to be a million I will never forget it. It's just bad. We tried using mints, which were somewhat effective, but not really. And it was one of those long-lasting things."

Some of these reactions are predictable, others are not. Always tell your chemotherapist or nurse of any sensations, no matter how silly they seem to you at the time. Occasionally the drug may leak into the surrounding tissue; this can be a serious side effect of chemotherapy, called *extravasation*. (See Chapter 12.)

THE FIRST TREATMENT

Some patients look forward to their first treatment because it signifies help for their disease. They are relieved that something can and is being done. Some experience an element of curiosity or excitement; many, however, approach their first "shot" with a good deal of anxiety and fear.

My doctor had warned me about vomiting and tiredness after a treatment, and that my hair might fall out later. These were only possibilities; I had no idea whether or not I would have them and this uncertainty was kind of exciting and horrifying at the same time. When the treatment was over, my husband and I rode the bus home. The anticipation was excruciating, but as the hours passed I only began to feel a little queasy and spaced-out, a little tired. That was all! Hardly the vision I had had of hanging out over the toilet bowl for hours. The next day, I still felt crummy, tired, and cranky.

Many people experience minimal side effects as I did; but the initial experiences vary, just as the overall experiences do:

"I was petrified to go for my first treatment. My doctor gave me the injection and had me lie down. Five minutes later he came back and asked, 'How are you feeling?' I felt fine and went home by subway alone, having sent my future husband Michael back to work. I thought if this is the way it's going to be, what's the big deal? About three hours later, I felt every ounce of energy drain from my body. My husband helped me get into bed and from that moment on I proceeded to throw up for four days."

"They started me on my first round of chemo while I was still in the hospital recovering from surgery. The resident on the case came in trundling a whole sack of little chemicals. Vile yellow colors, an ugly brown thing

... some of them were so-called antinausea drugs which knocked me out for the better part of the first day. That first day ... it was miserable. Feeling totally out of it, weak from the surgery, vomiting in spite of the antinausea drugs, my wife sort of floating in and out of my consciousness. My surgeon recommended that I hire a private duty nurse, and I thank God we had a health plan that allowed it—having someone there around the clock that first day really made a great deal of difference in my case."

"I thought: 'I'm going to go into this office and I'm going to see all these awful-looking people sitting around with all white faces.' I thought they would all be dying of cancer, and it would be depressing seeing all those people. But it didn't turn out like that at all."

"My doctor didn't tell me much about the side effects. So I wasn't terribly nervous—I didn't have that fear. When I started throwing up violently that night, I was frightened to death. I called him on the phone and said, 'If this is the way it's going to be every time, I can't go through with it!' It wasn't, though."

Since there's no way for you to know exactly what the initial chemo treatment is going to be like for you, the best course is to be as generally prepared as possible for every eventuality. Your preparation should include a basic grasp of what is going to happen before and during the injection, what will be expected of you, what the surroundings will be like, how long the injection will take, and what the immediate side effects might be. There is some dissension among the ranks as to how much detail a doctor should go into when describing the possible side effects of a particular set of drugs.

But if you are being treated as an outpatient, you should at least find out whether the side effects might affect your ability to get back home and function for the rest of the day. It is probably unwise in most cases to plan to put in a full day's— or evening's—activities after your injection. Though most drugs don't cause vomiting until hours after administration, and you may not feel any immediate effects at all, it is better to be safe than to be caught by surprise feeling sick in the middle of Main Street. In addition, you should be able to contact your doctor, or at least a knowledgeable nurse, in case anything occurs that you might need help with (as should be the case throughout your therapy).

Dr. Van Scoy-Mosher acknowledges that anxiety is a problem with some patients:

"What I've seen useful is for patients who are feeling particularly anxious to talk with another patient who had the same therapy. Patients can ask their doctors—I often arrange for this. Even if the patient had gotten sick with it—just to talk to somebody who had it a while ago or is having it and is still functioning, is doing okay, can relieve a lot of anxiety."

Donna Park, assistant director of Nursing, Ambulatory Care, at New York's Memorial Sloan-Kettering, says, "Most patients have absolutely no idea what chemotherapy means. When they come in for their first treatment, they're very frightened and apprehensive. They have no knowledge of how it's going to be given. They come in and they see a bottle hanging and they ask, 'What's that? I thought it was just a shot.'"

Many hospitals have instituted—or are in the throes of instituting—some kind of group orientation meetings for workshops to deal with the ins and outs of chemotherapy. While these can prepare you generally, they usually include a large variety of patients, cancers, and treatments, and so may not be specific enough. Your doctor or nurse is still the best source for nitty-gritty information about your chemotherapy plan. In addition, a patient volunteer—someone who has been through it—can share valuable firsthand experience. Your doctor, nurse, or hospital may also give you drug information cards which list the side effects and remedies, or other printed matter such as booklets, to reinforce whatever you have been told.

Ms. Park continues:

"Patients should have some knowledge, something in their hands, because they forget by the time they get home. They get bombarded with so much, and by the time they come for chemotherapy here, they're tired, they've been waiting for the doctor, the doctor has seen them, they may not like what was said to them, or the way it was said to them, they may have gotten bad news,

they may be worrying about the kids coming home from
school, or feeling angry . . . they're just not concentrating. They should have some form of written instruction."

Most oncologists advise against the patient's going alone
for any treatment, but this is especially important for the first
treatment, when the immediate side effects are more up in the
air than at any time during treatment. A familiar presence—a
spouse, parent, son or daughter, friend or neighbor—can allay
a lot of anxiety. He or she can also run interference, help deal
with red tape, ask questions for you, and perhaps retain more
information than you can at this time. From a purely practical
standpoint, another person can keep you company during long
waiting periods and accompany you home or take over any
driving that is necessary.

HANDLING THE SIDE EFFECTS

Without a doubt it is the side effects that have given chemotherapy a bad name and that worry people the most. Dr.
Richard Gralla feels that the media help paint an unfair view
of them. "People are misinformed, and some extra anxiety has
been built up because of that. A magazine article once said
that the cancer patient had to face the 'twin horrors' of cancer
and chemotherapy. That doesn't help people. A lot of things
have been done, especially in the last few years, to make the
side effects easier to take. Response to treatment can greatly
reduce the symptoms of cancer and bolster a person both physically and emotionally."

To a certain degree, your side effects can depend upon you—
your attitude and overall health—and upon your doctor. A
positive attitude, full of hope and confidence, can make side
effects less noticeable and more tolerable. A strong, healthy,
young body may withstand the rigors of some drugs better than
a weakened or older one. A good doctor-patient relationship
can make a contribution too: Sometimes it seems that the way
a patient feels about the oncologist has a great deal to do with
the severity of the side effects and how well the patient can
cope with them. In the hands of a competent, caring physician
or health care team, and with the judicious use of the support
services and therapies, the side effects picture is much better

than it used to be. Today, the side effects of chemotherapy are either preventable, treatable, of have the potential to be made more bearable.

Coping with side effects begins with an understanding of what they are, which ones you can reasonably expect to get, which ones are serious, and what you can do about them. Ideally, your oncologist will be able to help you in all these areas.

The science and art of medical oncology consist of treating the patient's cancer and treating the side effects caused by the treatment. Doing both well takes a lot of time and skill, as Dr. William Grace, chief of oncology at St. Vincent's Hospital in New York, explains:

> "Good care of patients is attention to detail. It's like anything else: If you are concerned about your patients you make every effort to assure that they don't get too sick from the disease or the therapy. Good care is labor-intensive, feeling compassion, having good ideas, and common sense. It means you have to do a lot of fine tuning. When the doctor-patient exchange is fruitful, medication can be given carefully and effectively in high doses without unacceptable toxicity."

No two people are exactly the same, and no two will react exactly the same to the same drugs, just as no two tumors will. The side effects that can be caused by the specific drugs in your chemotherapy plan are listed in the section that begins on page 277. A glance at this list can be terrifying and misleading—unless you remember this very important point: These are the side effects that *might* occur; they are not the ones that necessarily will occur. And, as you will see, there are many ways that you, your doctor, and your support system can work to prevent or alleviate those that do occur.

A few of the side effects listed for the drugs in your chemotherapy plan are very common and happen to some degree to nearly everyone who takes them; others are less common; and still others are quite rare. Side effects can sometimes occur in only a fraction of a percentage point of the total number of people who take the drugs. Some side effects may be only temporary or intermittent; or they may persist for the duration of the treatment, linger after treatment is just a memory, or never go away completely. They may be severe or slight, serious or minor, annoying or devastating. Sometimes there is confusion about whether a condition is actually the result of chemotherapy.

Oncologists are therefore put in a very tough position when their patients ask about side effects. People want to know what side effects they are going to get; they want to know what they can expect. Dr. Thomas Fahey of Memorial Sloan-Kettering in New York expresses the frustration of all oncologists when he says:

> "One of the things that's so frightening about it is that you can't sit down with a patient beforehand and say, 'Look, this is exactly what you're going to expect. And since this is what you can expect, this is what we're going to do about it.' It's so variable. I think it's probably not a good idea to present all the possible terrible things that can happen to people before they get chemotherapy because they may not get any of them. The patients should know, however, that certain side effects of chemotherapy are experienced to some degree by most patients who receive these treatments, and although they are variable, they are not unexpected. These could include stomach upset, hair loss, loss of energy, and blood count depression."

Dr. James A. Neidhart, chairman of the Department of Medical Oncology at the University of Texas System Cancer Center, M. D. Anderson Hospital and Tumor Institute, comments:

> "I don't volunteer information about very unusual side effects but I will answer questions I am asked. If you list all the possible side effects, you will scare a lot of people out of treatment. Is it fair to scare people out of treatment because of side effects that might affect one out of a thousand patients? We have more patients who decide not to accept effective treatment because they are unreasonably afraid of consent forms and side effects than we have patients who get into trouble because of side effects we haven't told them about. Secondly, 90 percent of my patients would fall asleep during the dis-

cussion. They don't want to know all the side effects; I can't even get through the routine side effects."

In addition, it is usually impossible to say exactly when side effects will occur and how long they will last. Some may occur within a few minutes or hours after the treatment. These include nausea and vomiting, extreme tiredness or weakness, dizziness, diarrhea, and constipation. These typically last a few hours to a few days, and then like a bad dream are over. In some cases, these side effects can plague the patient in milder form for some time. Often, a patient experiences a severe reaction with the very first treatment. In others, it can take many treatments until toxicity has built up. Reactions may be more severe after some treatments, almost negligible after others. Emotional states, too, can vary, with some reactions not taking hold for months until the reality and drudgery of chemotherapy sets in.

Dr. Fahey says:

"For some patients the hair loss is the worst possible thing that could ever be inflicted on them. Others, that doesn't bother at all. . . . It's the fact that they have to keep coming back to an institution or an office and being reminded that they have cancer. The chemotherapy is a continual reminder of the disease, the treatment must be given on a certain schedule, and their lives become so ordered around the schedule that that's the worst part of it. Then there are others who say they just feel crummy, that it makes them feel sick, nauseous. Some describe it as depression; I'm not sure it is a psychological depression, I think it's a physical depression. Chemotherapy depresses the whole body, and that's the most disturbing thing to them."

Sister Rosemary Moynihan, administrative supervisor in social work at Memorial Sloan-Kettering, says, "I find what really upsets people is prolonged nausea and vomiting, and weakness. Feeling tired, unattractive, not yourself, having no interest in anything. Even supermarket tabloids look too detailed for concentration."

For others, just the idea of chemotherapy is harder to cope with than the physical side effects. Sister Rosemary continues:

"I wouldn't underestimate the fear of 'it' coming into your body. The anger that that generates in some people! It's interesting—some people never get beyond the anger of chemo—they come in raging to every treatment. I think it's very difficult to have something injected into you that's alien to you. I think it makes most people feel very out of control. People talk about just the concept itself being a real problem. But you'd be crazy to dwell on it too much because sometimes it is the only option. And there are so many other things that you can dwell on that are a little more productive because you *can* do something about them, like buying pretty scarves or wigs if you lose your hair or working on your nutrition."

Your oncologist will be giving you tests and physical exams regularly to keep tabs on your condition. These tests, though bothersome, reveal valuable clues about what is going on inside your body and are an integral part of the chemotherapy treatment. Many of these tests—scans, X rays, lab tests—are also used during the initial diagnosis; during chemo, tests involving the blood are used with the greatest frequency and regularity.

Some of these tests reveal how well the drugs are working; others indicate how much damage is being done to normal cells (toxicity). Using the results of the tests, the oncologist decides whether to switch drugs, to increase the dosage, to decrease the dosage, to change the schedule, or to continue the therapy at all.

COMPLETE BLOOD COUNTS

Blood counts are the bread-and-butter tests of chemotherapy. The blood is composed of various types of cells which are produced in the bone marrow, spleen, and lymph glands. Both cancer and chemo can affect the composition of cells in your blood. A complete blood count (CBC) shows how your blood compares with the normal amounts of these cells and blood substances. Below are the normal amounts.

White blood cells fight infection (4,500–10,500).
Red blood cells, or erythrocytes, carry oxygen and waste (4.5–5 million).

Platelets, or thrombocytes, help clot the blood (200–350,000).

Hemoglobin is contained in the red cells and is responsible for carrying oxygen (13–16gm/100ml).

Hematocrit is the percentage of red blood cells (38–46 percent).

Differential is the ratio of mature cells to immature cells (100).

Your oncologist will order a CBC for you at least every time you are due for a treatment. Many oncologists feel that weekly tests are best, even if you don't have weekly treatments because real trends are more easily discernible the more data there is to go on, and because a low count may require attention immediately. Very low counts may require transfusions of blood products. If your count drops too low, your oncologist will hold back on your treatment, usually by reducing the dosage or by postponing the treatment.

Blood tests may be performed in your oncologist's office if there is a lab on the premises, or at a hospital, clinic, or independent laboratory. Blood may be drawn from a vein separately or through the intravenous needle used to administer chemotherapy if you are getting an IV drip and/or are being admitted as an inpatient to a hospital. Blood may also be taken from a finger prick—to spare veins for chemotherapy injections, oncologists sometimes order blood to be drawn only by this method.

After some time on chemo, I became adept at guessing when my blood count was down. I'd be feeling pretty down—tired, with no pep and gray face—and sure enough, it was down. So my doctor would pull back a bit on the drugs and I'd start to feel better. My count would creep up and he'd be able to blast away again. I think I found the blood tests more loathsome than the chemo injections. My technician had to use the finger prick each time because I had only one good vein in one good arm—the other arm was off-limits because of the mastectomy. She'd say "Ready?" and then make a quick jab and then squeeze and squeeze. I'd scrunch up my face each time; that somehow made it more tolerable. Between the blood tests every week and the chemo every other week, I felt like a pincushion. Over nine months of therapy, I was stuck a total of at least sixty times. In spite of all the jabbing, some patients manage to keep their senses of humor, as did this one who told me, "Every

Wednesday I had a blood test for lunch. I called the nurse my little vampire."

BIOCHEMISTRIES AND OTHER TESTS

The bulk of chemotherapy's side effects is due to toxicity to the rapidly reproducing cells in organs such as the blood-producing bone marrow. But, as Dr. Richard Gralla points out, "When you look closely at a variety of drugs, it's not the bone marrow that is the major limitation, it's other organs." This second group of vital organs includes the lungs, heart, liver, kidney, bladder, and nerves. Damage to these organs may be quick, dramatic, and difficult to predict, or slow, insidious, and easy to miss. Sometimes these organs need to be pushed only a little before the damage becomes irreversible. The danger to these organs may be great or small, depending upon the drugs, the doses, and the health of the organs to begin with. New drugs and high doses pose especially high risks. Your oncologist will order tests to monitor the condition of these organs if you fall into the high-risk category.

In Adriamycin, for example, the dose-limiting toxicity (the side effect that limits the amount of drug that can be safely given) occurs to the heart; in cisplatinum, the kidneys and auditory nerves are in jeopardy; in the nitrosureas, the kidneys and lungs may be damaged; high doses of cytoxan can affect the heart. The danger of harming these organs is why it is necessary to give tests such as EKGs or echocardiogram for the heart, hearing tests, blood chemistry tests, liver function tests, and pulmonary functions tests periodically, and sometimes daily for a period of time.

BIOLOGICAL MARKERS

Biological markers (also called tumor markers) are substances that either are contained within cancer cells or are released by them into the bloodstream. Some of these are chemicals that normally occur in the body but whose levels are higher when cancer is present. A few of these tests have become fairly standard. Many more have recently been developed and are being tested. So far, none of these tests is perfect. They are not foolproof in detecting all types of cancer with 100 percent accuracy. Specific tests are limited in their abilities to detect specific cancers, and their accuracy rates are 87 percent or less. Though they are not the last word, they do represent exciting new tools in monitoring and detecting cancer growth and regression, especially in the early detection of recurrences or metastases. Among the alphabet soup of biological markers for which your blood may be tested are: CEA, AFP, SCM, MEM, TPA, B-protein, BCFP, CMA, SCAP, GT-II, POA, ZGM.

But lab tests and physical exams are only one component of the ongoing monitoring process. It also consists of the feedback you give your oncologist. Doctors and their nurses should be accessible and willing and able to give you the time you need, but they are not mind readers.

When your doctor asks you how you feel, be honest. You might fib to your friends and family if you feel it's necessary to put up a good front, but you should never lie to your oncologist about your condition. Don't say you feel fine when you feel lousy. It is not your responsibility to make him or her feel good and be pleased with your condition. It is your responsibility to do all in your power to help your oncologist help you; help cannot be forthcoming if he or she hasn't a clue. Bravery can make you very sick, so don't tell your doctor what you think your doctors wants to hear—tell what he or she needs to hear.

The sooner you report a side effect, the sooner it can be treated. Even if it's not "serious," there's no reason you should suffer even the slightest unnecessary discomfort, worry, or danger. In addition, what seems unimportant or insignificant to you could lead to something serious or be an indication of other already serious troubles.

Dr. Michael Van Scoy-Mosher says:

"There's no question that patients are very symptom-conscious. I think one thing the physician can do is make the patients feel welcome to call with what they know are often minor complaints. One minute on the phone can sometimes head off two weeks of anxiety.

"Sometimes when patients call up with certain complaints, I try to explain to them why I don't think that's important. I don't just say, 'Don't worry about it.' It depends upon the patient—for instance, if he or she has a backache today, and tomorrow the shoulder aches a little bit, and next week the rib aches, that's not something to worry about."

Many side effects can indeed wait until you see your doctor or nurse during your next scheduled treatment. Some, however, may indicate that you are seriously ill and should be treated right away.

I have included a list of possible signs of the side effects that can be serious enough to require immediate treatment. If you are unsure, or worried, speak up instantly. Speak to the doctor or nurse on the phone; if possible your problem may be able to be settled right then and there. If not, your doctor might want you to make an appointment or to admit you to a hospital. If you cannot reach your doctor, you can get in touch with the physician who is covering for him or her. As a last resort, you can go to the emergency room of the nearest hospital to which your doctor has admitting privileges or to the hospital at which you are receiving treatment as an outpatient. Not all cancer centers have emergency rooms, and clinics do not have inpatients at all. If you do go to a hospital with which your oncologist is not affiliated, he cannot treat you while you are there; you will be treated by a staff or house physician.

SIDE EFFECTS THAT SHOULD BE REPORTED IMMEDIATELY

- Fever over 100 degrees Fahrenheit
- Bleeding or bruising
- Rash or other allergic reaction (swollen eyelids, hands, feet)
- Shaking and chills
- Pain at the injection site
- Unusual pain anywhere, including headaches and joint pain
- Shortness of breath
- Severe diarrhea or constipation
- Bloody urine

Your oncologist has several approaches available to alleviate the side effects you may develop. One is to change the timing or the way chemo is given—this works for a few side effects such as nausea, tiredness, phlebitis, and heart toxicity. A recent study showed that there was much less toxicity when cisplatin is given in the evening rather than the morning, and when adriamycin was given in the morning rather than the evening. Another option might be to suggest nondrug therapies such as nutrition, exercise, and psychological therapy or counseling. (See Chapters 8, 9, and 15). A third approach is to reduce the dosage or frequency of treatment. This course is usually taken only if the side effect is serious—that is, life threatening—such as a low blood count as opposed to nausea, and if no other effective method exists to relieve it. The last tactic, to prescribe additional symptom-relieving medication, is sometimes preferred when the other methods are ineffective or because reducing the chemo drugs reduces the drugs' effectiveness to too great a degree. (Doctors may, of course, use any combination of these methods.) Fortunately, medication usually works just as well on conditions caused by chemo as on those due to some other reason.

Medication is useful, for instance, in controlling pain that might otherwise ruin your sleep, your appetite, and your social life. If you are nauseous and vomiting, an antinausea drug may help you maintain a better nutritional status and boost your morale. Insomnia can wear you out, but the short-term use of sleeping pills will help you get the rest you need to face the next day and help your body to replace the tissue being damaged by chemotherapy. If you are depressed or anxious about your disease and its treatment, a tranquilizer or antidepressant can help restore your sense of well-being and relieve stress that may be detrimental to your prognosis and your quality of life.

Drugs such as these can bring welcome relief, but they can also impose their own set of distressing side effects. They may not; but if they do, these in turn can be treated. For instance, narcotics used to control pain often cause constipation which in turn can be alleviated by laxatives, enemas, stool softeners, and a change in the diet. Antinausea medication is usually sedative, but this can be dealt with by changing the schedule of medication.

Though it is generally wise to keep any additional drugs to a minimum, and some people may prefer to try nondrug methods first, drugs do have their uses. Just as strong drugs are needed to fight cancer, other drugs may at some point be justified to keep us going. When symptoms are severe, acute, or don't respond well enough to nondrug measures, the stress and discomfort caused by the unrelieved symptom may be more harmful than the drug that relieves it. It is reasonable to be concerned about drugs you don't need, but drastic times call for drastic measures and you shouldn't hesitate to call upon modern medicine for help. Part of living with cancer entails living in the here and now—and not being overly concerned with what a drug might do in some undefined future. The benefits of taking additional medication, especially if it's temporary, may far outweigh the risks.

I had a prescription for Compazine, but I never took it. My nausea wasn't bad and I figured since I was being pumped up with all those other drugs, why take more unless I really had to? I did eventually take something for a week or so to help me get to sleep. And then I also took an antidepressant for about a month. But it made me feel dizzy, so I stopped. By that time I was over the big depression anyway. As my doctor said, "We have to use whatever we need to get you through this."

Dr. William Grace, for another, believes that you should "use whatever pharmacology you have to so a patient may lead as normal a life as possible." He notes that some of his patients have discovered that Dexatrim counteracts some of the fatigue related to chemo; some doctors even prescribe Dexedrine for this same purpose in selected patients. He says:

"You have to remember that in small, careful doses, it's safe, and that chemotherapy patients are not drug abusers—they are quite normal people for whom a little bit of Dexedrine goes a long way. These people don't easily become drug dependent. When they finish the chemotherapy course, they don't want any more Dexedrine, or other medicines that made the therapy more tolerable."

You should be aware that both over-the-counter (OTC) and prescription drugs can affect you more than usual or interact dangerously with chemotherapy drugs. Common aspirin, for example, can compound the problem of slow blood clotting. Chemotherapy patients are usually advised to switch to aspirin-free analgesics and to learn to read labels carefully since many OTC products contain aspirin. Even diuretics and antibiotics can interact with your chemotherapy regimen.

Always inform your chemotherapist of any drugs you may

be taking and keep him up-to-date on any changes. Other drugs that may interfere with chemotherapy include: anticoagulants, blood pressure drugs, anticonvulsants, barbiturates, cough medicines, sleeping pills, tranquilizers, and birth control pills.

Alcohol is not usually thought of as a drug, but it *is* one, so some thought should be given to its use during chemotherapy. Usually, the chemotherapy patient is able to drink some alcohol—one or two glasses of wine or beer a day. Occasionally, however, no alcohol is allowed because it can aggravate the side effects of some drugs. In addition, consumption of huge amounts of alcohol can cause liver damage and vitamin deficiencies. Not only can chemotherapy cause the same to happen, but a well-functioning liver is crucial in detoxifying the anticancer drugs, so be sure to ask your doctor about alcohol consumption. I'm not exactly a lush, but I do like wine when I go out. When I asked if wine was permissible, my doctor said, "Sure, go ahead, have some fun." But I began to notice that even a glass or two made me more tired the next day. I was feeling tired enough from my chemo, so I stopped the booze altogether. Later, my surgeon told me this was quite common.

Other common medical measures that may be called upon to support the chemotherapy patient and limit the short- and long-term effects include the various blood products. When the blood count falls too low, transfusions of red cells, platelets, or leukocytes may be required together or individually. Bone marrow transplants, though still considered experimental, are coming in use. Leucovorin rescue is a procedure used that enables patients to withstand huge doses of Methotrexate without harming the healthy cells. In this technique, the Methotrexate is followed by another drug Leucovorin which protects or "rescues" normal cells from the Methotrexate's life-threatening toxic effects.

When drugs fail to relieve pain, or their side effects are unacceptable, there are medical alternatives: neurosurgery on nerves that transmit the pain or surgery on local pain blocks.

TREATING THE WHOLE PERSON

There is more to progressive, caring chemotherapy than simply giving a passive patient the right anticancer drugs in the right amounts, and there is more to minimizing side effects than supplying patients with yet more drugs. Though a sound, disease-oriented treatment is paramount and symptom-relieving drugs have their place, a disease cannot be treated completely and humanely in isolated technological splendor. It is becoming increasingly obvious that since the chemo patient is affected totally, he or she needs to be treated as a whole person. Medicine, in the narrow sense of using drugs to treat disease, cannot begin to determine and fulfill the patient's physical, psychological, social, and spiritual needs, but broadening its scope to include nondrug support therapies can. "Good medicine" can help you keep your life at the highest quality possible, by taking care of the rest of you while the chemo takes care of the cancer.

The next few chapters include suggestions for a wide variety of steps you can take and methods you can utilize to get through chemotherapy as unscathed as possible. They include emotional help from family, friends, and professionals; stress management and reduction; diet and nutrition; and exercise. Which ones you choose, to what degree you utilize them, where you find them, and how they fit in with your chemotherapy program depends upon your individual reactions to chemotherapy, your needs, your style, and your own resources. For some patients these therapies play a major and integral part in keeping body and soul together.

My oncologist, who looks to both traditional and non-traditional sources of support for his cancer patients, believes:

"The most important thing in medicine is to individualize. Each person needs something slightly different. You can't just use the cookie cutter system. An oncologist has to use the very finest that is available at the present time. That includes a continuing search for protocols that have been demonstrated to be of validity in doses that have been shown to be valuable; it includes very careful attention to the known side effects and known toxic effects of the medication; and it includes their application in a program that involves a certain amount of building and strengthening of the body as well as simply destroying."

Through all your emotional and physical experiences, your oncologist is the central figure around whom everything else seems to revolve. Your doctor, then, is the most natural person to whom you turn for support. In an ideal world, he or she would be able to treat all your related needs or to recommend people who can. In reality, doctors are somewhat limited in their methods and patients often look elsewhere for help—to a primary-care physician or nurse, or to someone outside the medical mainstream. Always inform your oncologist of any additional therapies you are undertaking. Make it clear at the outset that they are being used as supplementary therapies to, not in place of, chemotherapy. Even if your oncologist does not endorse a particular therapy (chances are getting better that he or she will), it is important to reveal everything there is to know about your health practices. Some—such as the more extreme diets—may actually do more harm than good. But if a therapy does do good, the information may be passed on to other patients.

When used as supplements to chemotherapy, support therapies can be thought of as a form of "insurance" and a means of improving the quality of life that is being eroded by the drugs. In addition, these therapies can help to fill the gap between the cold technical approach sometimes offered the patient, and the warm, human approach the patient really needs. Perhaps their greatest value, however, lies in the way they enable you to play a more active role in your treatment, to feel a sense of control rather than playing the part of a passive patient leaving your life totally in the hands of the doctor and the drugs. Chemotherapy need not be a spectator sport. Dr. Ernest Rosenbaum writes in the introduction of his book, *A Comprehensive Guide for Cancer Patients and Their Families*:

> "When you are an active participant in your medical care and rehabilitation, you can maintain a sense of control over your disease and your therapy. Only you can take responsibility for your state of mind, nutritional status, and physical fitness. The act of taking responsibility is in itself an important factor in maintaining self-esteem, a feeling of independence, and faith in your ability to cope. It is a critical part of therapy."

CHAPTER 6

Emotional Help

Beginning with the diagnosis and continuing throughout and after treatment, cancer patients need to make many psychological adjustments. Your new life has brought with it both intangible emotional reactions and concrete problems. Though many patients (and their families) do manage to somehow cope well enough on their own, there is no reason not to call upon the many services and therapies that have been designed to make the coping process easier. Some people believe that anything that helps reduce stress may also extend the life of a cancer patient.

Like the other support services for cancer patients, the field of *psychosocial oncology*, which deals with the way the patient and family react to the disease and its treatment, is fairly new. Grace Christ, the director of social work at New York's Memorial Sloan-Kettering and editor of the *Journal of Psychosocial Oncology*, says, "It's taken time for people to appreciate some of the psychosocial consequences of cancer and its treatments. But as cancer patients live longer and the disease becomes long-term or chronic, or one from which people are cured, the social and emotional effects become much more visible." Psychosocial support services exist in several forms— individual work, group work, family work, and multiple family work.

94

The idea of emotional counseling for the cancer patient has met with resistance from professionals and patients alike. On the patient's side, old taboos die hard: There is still some stigma attached to admitting that you might need a little help with your emotional problems. A social worker told me:

"People tend, in our culture especially, to underappreciate the impact of the disease and the treatment. We tend to be a bit stoical in general and don't really understand how much we're being affected. Talking to someone, or using some outside help, doesn't mean we're weak, it doesn't mean we're coping poorly. It means we'd like to cope better, and this is one way to do that. Most people manage to cope reasonably well. But sometimes you can cope better and your whole experience can be of a different quality."

Lari Wenzel, former director of the Cancer Information Service at the Comprehensive Cancer Center for the state of Florida says:

"It is not unusual for people to have a need for support services during a time that is particularly stressful, regardless of what that stress is. Cancer as a chronic disease introduces particular stressors to the individual's life. Even people who normally handle stress well can use a little help with problems that may arise as a result of this diagnosis."

Your oncologist, family doctor, or nurse should be able to help you and your family get over some of the hurdles you will face, and perhaps all of them. However, physicians are often unaware of their patients' need for emotional support. In addition, most doctors and nurses are not trained as counselors or therapists. You may find yourself turning elsewhere for additonal emotional support.

When shopping around for emotional assistance, be as choosy as when looking for medical help. Some professionals are more skilled or have had more experience with cancer patients than others, and some approaches may be more comfortable for you than others.

One bad or unproductive experience should not discourage

you or prevent you from seeking another more understanding or suitable source of therapy, as happened in my case.

The only person I spoke to about my cancer was the Reach to Recovery lady who just popped into my hospital room a few days after the mastectomy. She was so stiff and formal, I couldn't identify with her at all. She just left me a ball, a booklet, a bra, and a boob made out of polyester. Sure, she wore a tight sweater to let me know that it is possible to look "normal" after a mastectomy. But she came before I was really ready to see anyone; I was still too shocked to think straight and ask questions. When I visited the Reach to Recovery office to look at prostheses, they were so grim about the whole thing . . . maybe I'm nuts, but I saw some humor in opening up a whole filing cabinet drawer full of breasts. I wanted to talk to someone, but I knew I didn't want to talk to *them*. So I ended up not talking to anybody.

Grace Christ feels that "People should not hesitate to seek help. I think it can't hurt, even if it is just to stabilize yourself. But it's not always as accessible as it should be." Part of the problem, she feels, is that in the past, people tended to think that support for cancer patients was either straight education— giving information—or intensive psychotherapy. Though it can include both of these, today psychosocial support comes in a wide variety of flavors (or "interventions"). Whatever your taste and your needs, there is something for you, be it traditional psychotherapy, self-help groups, or anything in between. Sometimes one or two sessions with a social worker will point the way for your problem solving, or a chat with a patient volunteer will help to put things in perspective and your mind at ease.

Reputable sources for emotional help include your physician, nurses, hospital social workers, psychologists, psychiatrists, county health departments, neighborhood mental health clinics, and the various national, regional, and local cancer support organizations listed in the back of the book, such as the American Cancer Society and the Cancer Information Service.

PSYCHOTHERAPY

Sometimes it is helpful to talk, one-on-one, with someone who can be objective and nonjudgmental, and who is knowledgeable about cancer and experienced in helping others work out their feelings. When this need arises, there are psychiatrists, psychologists, nurse-clinicians, and psychiatric social workers who specialize in treating people with cancer.

Psychotherapy can prove valuable in some cases—dealing with cancer and chemotherapy can exacerbate present personality problems, or resurrect old ones. However, most patients do not require or want long-term therapy. There are easier, less intense, less protracted, less expensive, more specific, and more appropriate forms of therapy to fulfill the chemotherapy patient's combined needs for education, practical resources, and psychosocial support. "Crisis intervention" is a short-term therapy specifically designed to get you through a tough time. Dr. Judith Bukberg, a psychiatrist at St. Vincent's Hospital in New York, who specializes in treating cancer patients, says, "It's important to understand the difference between counseling and therapy. Counseling is largely a directive, supportive interaction. Therapy is not. Therapy is exploratory. It tries to figure out why something's going on."

SOCIAL WORKERS

Social workers serve a wide variety of functions in our society but, unfortunately, are usually thought of in terms of the welfare system. Medical social workers, however, are the mainstay of the medical system in helping cancer patients and their families find ways to get through it all. In their basic roles of troubleshooters/problem solvers, social workers can help you grasp the realities of living on chemotherapy and work to improve those areas over which you have some control. To that end, they will familiarize themselves with your problems and concerns and work with you to take care of them, be they medical, financial, emotional, religious, or related to your family or employment situation. Social workers can help you communicate with the medical system, help you slice through red tape, and help you and your family work together to detect and meet any emotional or practical needs. They can provide or help find useful items like wheelchairs, prostheses, bedpans, bandages, and financial assistance if you need them. Social workers can help you fill out forms, organize your time around your treatment schedule, arrange for housekeepers, child care, housing, or hospice service. And since there are psychiatric social workers who are specially trained in this field, they can provide psychotherapy when emotional problems appear to keep you from functioning as well as you might.

Social workers often engage in individual counseling with patients alone, with patients and their families, or with families alone. They also either run support groups or can put you in touch with support groups near your home. Every hospital has social workers, but their availability and usefulness vary. If you need help, a good way to start is to contact a staff social worker at your community hospital or the hospital where you are being treated and see to what extent that person meets your needs.

SUPPORT GROUPS

Support groups have an overwhelming advantage over other forms of support in that they consist of other people like you who have cancer. Because of this common bond, many people feel more relaxed and find it easier to communicate with other cancer patients than with their families, friends, doctors, or nurses. "Because it reduces anxiety," says Ms. Christ, "this kind of group is often the kind of forum in which people hear most easily." Many patients and professionals agree that a group is an ideal environment to exchange experiences and methods of dealing with both the practical and emotional issues surrounding cancer and its treatment.

Sister Rosemary Moynihan, a social worker at Memorial Sloan-Kettering in New York City, also points out:

"Groups help patients to make the decision to accept therapy, to continue it, to change it, to stop it. They help patients fill in gaps in their information, or correct misinformation. We often try to help patients clarify their thoughts when they may be having trouble putting them into words."

However, another social worker observes: "Many people are shy of groups and given an option would avoid them. But once they get started they find it's something that's very useful." Patients who participate in support groups say they sleep better, are less depressed, and feel more comfortable talking about their illness. For example:

"The night after the first meeting, I went home and slept like a baby—fourteen, fifteen hours—better than I'd slept in a long time. I'd talked to people who understood. At first I thought it would be a waste of time, but it was very comforting. Now that I belong to a group, I can let out my feelings without burdening my friends with my concerns. I wish I had joined one earlier—I was one and a half years into cancer. I went through all those things you go through alone."

"I think it's better to talk to other people who are having chemo because the doctor doesn't know how you feel. If you talk to patients, they have the same problems as you."

"It's so good to talk to somebody who's been through it and is living a normal life again. I was so afraid of losing my hair, losing too much weight, not being able to take care of my children."

Support groups can help you keep or regain your self-esteem, your balance, and your self-worth. A good support group is made up of people who believe in each other, who offer each other optimistic, realistic help, encouragement, stimulation, meaningful advice, and valuable connections. When you belong to a group, you get help and give it too.

However, the whole idea of baring your innermost thoughts in front of a group of people may not be your style, or it may not be helpful. And it may be difficult to find the right group, as this patient comments:

"The doctor got four of us together. It was nice in a way because I walked in feeling I was the only person in the world who had to wear a wig, and here were these two other girls in wigs looking perfectly normal. But part of it was depressing. One of them was only twenty-one years old and I found it difficult to deal with somebody that young going through this. She was getting a more difficult chemo than I was—it really broke my heart; I really felt for her."

Dr. Ward F. Cunningham-Rundles, an oncologist at Memorial Sloan-Kettering in New York, finds that groups may not be the answer for everyone:

"One certainly has to have some kind of personal interaction; if people don't mesh, then they don't mesh. They have to be the *right* people too. If you're in a protocol that causes you to be affected in a different way from the others in the group—if there are other patients with a very poor prognosis and one by one they do poorly, that can be difficult to take."

The quality of the groups and the degree to which they are helpful vary depending upon the input of the members and the experience and leadership capabilities of the organizers. Support groups are not "therapy" groups—they are coping groups. They are work-oriented; the most useful groups tend to focus on rehabilitation—the process of adjusting to the disease and its treatment and getting back into life. Groups that resemble mere gripe sessions have their uses but tend to have their limitations. As Sister Rosemary says, "You need someone to lead the group, to keep the discussion going, to protect the members, to see that the information being relayed is appropriate and correct."

Support groups take a variety of forms. They may be very heterogeneous with patients having different cancers, prognoses, ages, disease stages, and family situations, or they may be more homogeneous and composed of people with the same disease, such as breast cancer or Hodgkin's disease; they may involve patients receiving the same form of treatment or those in a specific age group. These groups might meet only with patients, or the family, or with both. They often include trained patient volunteers and are usually led by one or more professionals such as social workers, psychotherapists, psychiatric nurses, or members of the clergy. Self-help groups are a breed of support groups that are organized by cancer patients themselves; some are local chapters of national organizations.

Alternatives to support groups exist that might suit your needs better. These are trained volunteers, some of them patients themselves, whom you can meet with personally or are just a phone call away. Your hospital or physician or community cancer organization can put you in touch with a trained volunteer, or you have access to an empathetic ear via the cancer hotlines scattered across the country, as this patient did:

"Unless you have gone through the same type of situation, or are very close to someone who has, you just don't have the empathy, you don't understand. We have nobody to talk to. The day I called the Kansas City Hotline, I was crying, I was feeling so sorry for myself. But the woman I spoke to was so warm—and she was a living statistic. It made me feel so good. It cost me twelve dollars—we talked a long time—but it was worth every dime of it."

I wish I had been as smart as this patient. I think if I had just talked to even one other person who had had or who was having chemotherapy, I wouldn't have felt as terrified or as alone as I did at times. I wish I had thought of it, or that my oncologist had suggested it, instead of mentioning psychiatrists; but we didn't.

FAMILY AND FRIENDS

Studies have shown that people who have strong relationships or support systems—whether family or friends—usually do better than those who go through it alone. Lari Wenzel, who has found this to be true in her own experience, adds that "support groups help, but they can't completely take the place of those with whom you have an established relationship."

In his book *Living with Cancer*, Dr. Ernest Rosenbaum points out that as the traditional concept of the passive patient is becoming old hat, so is the idea that the family is an outside element. Both patient and family, or close friends, are able to contribute immeasurably to cancer care. He writes: "Having the family 'wait outside' wastes a great deal of valuable energy that could be available as additional 'people power' to facilitate a patient's recovery. Also, many family members need to do something to actively contribute to the patient's getting-well process."

How the family handles the crisis of cancer and chemotherapy usually depends upon how well the family has functioned in the past. Good relationships often get even better; many cancer patients report a learning, growing experience that brings them closer to their spouses, other family members, and friends.

You can let friends and family know when their help is welcome in practical matters such as child care, cooking, shopping, phone calls, housework, and other errands and domestic chores. They can encourage healthful activities and low-key diversions such as taking a walk, going for a drive, taking in a movie, museum, or play, and visiting others, or—keeping your physical limitations in mind—more strenuous activities such as swimming or bike riding. They can improve your sense of well-being through massage. They can act as researchers— by asking questions, writing letters, or going to the library— if you want additional information about your disease and its treatment.

Loved and loving family members often provide moral support and the motivation to continue treatment when one's own will falters:

> "Sometimes I didn't want to go for the chemo. Just as I was getting my system back together, it was time to go back for another treatment. My twenty-one year-old daughter was with me through it all. When I got a little weak and didn't want to go, that little stinker said, 'You'd better go and have those treatments because if I ever got breast cancer and I needed chemo, I'd go. But if you don't finish your treatments, Mom, I'm not going either.' Blackmail! But she kept me going."

> "I don't know how many nights I spent sitting on the floor in the bathroom, my head bent over the toilet bowl, my husband patting my head, and my saying to him, 'I'm quitting it. I've had enough. I don't need it. I don't want it.' I might have quit, too, if I didn't have someone there stroking me saying, 'You're going to be okay. You're going to see this through. You know you can. You know you have to.'"

Family members can help by accompanying you to the facility when you go for a checkup or a treatment. Having someone come along during a question-and-answer session or during a treatment is a simple yet important step in their understanding the treatment and in lending their support.

Sometimes I'd feel so alone and vulnerable sitting in my doctor's waiting room, and later on the bus ride home, that I'd ask Michael to come with me. It wasn't that I felt sick after my shot or that I couldn't get home on my own. Sometimes I was just frightened and it felt good just having him there, holding my hand, or just reading magazines together while we waited. Once a friend asked me if I wanted her to go with me. I knew she was torn up over my having cancer and hated the fact that she couldn't do anything about it. I think she was just plain curious about the chemo, too. So even though it didn't make the cancer or the chemo go away, she came along. She felt better and so did I.

And yet obstacles often prevent family and friends from living up to their full potential as helpers—the patient won't let them, or they don't know how, or they are having too much trouble coping themselves to help the patient cope. There may be some difficulty in discussing the illness, the treatment, and the prognosis. There may be a reluctance to face the unpleasant or a desire to protect each other. (Cancer patients have said that a lack of communication within the family is one of the major problems they face in coping with their disease and its treatment.) Cancer and its treatment cause massive shifts in responsibilities, roles, and life patterns in addition to emotional upheavals. It is tempting for the family to focus exclusively on the patient's disease, so that friendships fade away and hobbies and interests fall by the wayside. Or people may feel that since the patient is in the hands of the doctors, there is nothing they can do. Patients may have trouble juggling the desire to assert their independence with the real need for help and the desire to let others feel useful.

Some families are able to solve their own problems and adapt to the new situation easily. But many others could benefit from some kind of assistance in adjusting to the new reality before they can effectively help each other. If help is not offered, and you feel you and your family could use some assistance in getting back on the right track, ask for it. Meeting with your oncologist, oncology nurse, a social worker, a family therapist, or a family-oriented support group can make great strides in educating your family unit, helping its members to communicate and sort out their feelings and realize they are normal, and encouraging them to develop their own coping strategies.

RELIGION AND THE CLERGY

In times of trouble, religion is a refuge for many, be it drawn upon privately in the form of meditation and prayer, or more publicly in the form of support and guidance from the clergy and/or fellow members of the congregation. A strong belief system can be a source of hope and comfort to a person who is undergoing treatment for cancer, as this patient says: "I had a lot of help because I have a lot of faith. There's a psalm that goes 'Lift up your eyes into the hills from whence cometh my help. My help cometh from the Lord.' And oh, that verse really took me through it."

Severe stress may lead some people to revert to discarded religious beliefs. Even when patients no longer have any religious affiliation or are not about to return to the fold, a member of the clergy—of no matter what faith—can still be a welcome, sympathetic figure. It is part of a clergyman's job and training to comfort the sick and troubled, to encourage people to unburden their souls. Members of the clergy can be very good listeners, and the trappings of religion aside, just having someone who is interested, who understands, and who has time for you can be very good for the soul.

CHAPTER 7

Stress Management and Reduction

Many attempts have been made to correlate personality, attitude, and stress with the onset and course of an illness such as cancer. Although some of these studies have been more successful than others, the overall results of such studies are far from conclusive. However, many researchers are turning up evidence that does link psychological states in humans with the efficacy of the immune system in general and with the development and progress of cancer specifically.

According to these studies, positive states of mind such as feelings of happiness, independence, control over life, and relaxation tend to keep the immune system going strong and perhaps even strengthen an immune system that has been weakened (as it is by chemotherapy). Negative states of mind—feelings of hopelessness, helplessness, depression, passivity, or anxiety—influence hormone production that could further debilitate a chemotherapy-weakened immune system and make it less capable of combating an already established cancer, and more susceptible to the infectious diseases to which a chemotherapy patient is prone.

There is clearly a very complex link between the brain and the body, and it is barely understood. Those who practice anticancer therapies based on solely this connection are on scientifically shaky ground. The advocates of these therapies assert, however, that perhaps everything in this world cannot be explained according to today's scientific precepts. In any event, the other values of these therapies cannot be ignored.

Barbara Blumberg, a public health educator with the National Cancer Institute's Cancer Information Service, says:

> "You can poke holes in every single study that's been done equating cancer with some emotionally stressful situation. On the other hand, people think enough of the studies that have been done that they are trying to replicate them and learn more. As far as attitudes being able to help chemotherapy patients—that's a whole other story. This does not have to be based on scientific evidence, but on common sense: If your attitude is better about going on these drugs, chances are you're going to be more compliant and have more chance of them working."

A positive attitude, a will to live, optimism, and a fighting spirit are crucial elements in your treatment. Even though the part they play in actually fighting cancer may be relatively minor, the part they play in your desire and ability to tolerate debilitating treatment may be major. A positive outlook which makes you feel more relaxed and in control will improve the quality of your life, no matter how much time you have left. How much better it is to face everything with hope and equanimity than with helplessness and despair.

WHAT YOU CAN DO ABOUT STRESS

Basically there are two things you can do to relieve stress. First, you can try to remove as much stress as possible. Second, you can try to learn how to deal with the necessary stress in a positive way. In order to accomplish either of these tasks, you must first be able to discern exactly what it is that is creating the stress. Sometimes just becoming aware of stress can begin to help; then you take it seriously and figure out ways to deal with it. Saying you are afraid of "cancer" or "chemotherapy" is not specific enough. For instance, if you are overly concerned about your prognosis, speak to your doctor who may be able to assuage your anxieties. If you are afraid of being alone during treatments or afterward, ask a family member or close friend to stay with you. If you feel uncomfortable because you've lost all your hair, make the effort to find a natural-looking wig.

Emotional counseling, discussed in the previous chapter, is another avenue to explore. With professional guidance, you can begin to fight back. Instead of bottling up frustrations and tensions and leaving them to bubble up inside, letting them out and letting go can reduce the harm that chronic tension can do. And you can help your body withstand stress better by maintaining general health—getting adequate nutrition, avoiding cigarettes, limiting coffee and alcohol intake and other drugs, and getting enough rest and exercise.

Another way to cope with stress is through specific stress management/reduction techniques. Eastern medicine and philosophy have long recognized that the mind and the body are one and that people have the potential to control their minds and through them their bodies. This interrelationship between mind and body and the techniques used to exploit it have only recently begun to be appreciated by Western medicine. Though these techniques can be used by anyone, many of them are now being developed specifically and used as adjuvant treatments to relieve the physical and emotional side effects of cancer and chemotherapy.

These techniques, which range from simple relaxation methods to more advanced "mind-control" practices, include biofeedback, meditation, controlled deep breathing, progressive muscle relaxation, self-hypnosis, and creative imagery or visualization. Therapists usually combine two or more into a unique package, in accordance with their style, training and preferences, and the requirements and abilities of the patient. Often the simpler techniques serve as stepping stones for the more advanced methods. (In addition, there may be a psychotherapeutic element involved.)

Matthew Loscalzo, a social worker at Memorial Sloan-Kettering in New York, who is trained in these techniques, stresses the importance of using an integrated approach:

"Some people feel that self-hypnosis is a strong enough tool to use by itself to reach many goals. I do not share that view. I never do only one thing: Hypnotherapy is only part of my overall treatment plan. The issues going on are much too important and complex. We need to make our treatments at least as complex as our patients."

Regardless of the name or level, such techniques are all based upon the ability of the mind to directly control many of the bodily processes that Western medicine has traditionally thought to be involuntary. Traditional medical doctors tend to have trouble with this concept, even those who accept the results of studies that show that placebos (sugar pills) work 20 to 40 percent of the time. If a placebo works because the mind, which believes in the medicine, actually brings about the expected effect, why can't these techniques work this way too? Experiments at the Menninger Clinic have shown that it is possible for someone to control *a single nerve cell* through biofeedback techniques.

Faith in their efficacy and willingness to throw aside preconceived notions seem to be key elements in using these techniques effectively. M. L. Frohling, a biofeedback technician and part of the oncology team at Denver Presbyterian Hospital, says:

> "To make visualization/biofeedback/relaxation effective, you have to really believe in the major underlying principle that mind and body act as a unit. You have a particular thought or image and that's going to elicit a physiological response. You can envision sucking on a lemon and you will respond to that image: You will taste the tartness and start to salivate. But you have to have a really deep belief for that to happen."

These techniques, in principle and in practice, strike people used to Western ways of thinking and doing as wild or weird—they take time to learn, to use, and to show results. We don't know exactly why or how they work; they do not work for everyone, or to the same extent. But in many cases where drugs have failed to work their magic, and without adding any harmful side effects of their own, these techniques are achieving results in reducing stress and controlling symptoms and side effects of cancer and chemotherapy. They have successfully reduced or eliminated anxiety, tension, insomnia, nausea, vomiting, diarrhea, lethargy, depression, feelings of helplessness and hopelessness, and pain in chemotherapy patients. They have increased patients' feelings of well-being, relaxation, and control over their lives.

BIOFEEDBACK

When you are under stress, your body reacts in several ways—muscles tense up, blood vessels constrict, blood pressure goes up, hand temperature goes down, and so on. Biofeedback (short for biological feedback) is a way of measuring and monitoring these bodily processes and feeding this information back to you visually or aurally so you can see or hear it. But having a direct line to your physiological responses is only a beginning. While you are hooked up to the machinery, the idea is to learn how to follow its signals and thus voluntarily change them.

Unless you know specific relaxation techniques to effect these changes, you learn to relax by trial and error, a process that takes considerable time, effort and patience. M. L. Frohling, for example, puts patients on biofeedback machines as a first step in her total therapeutic package, which utilizes a combination of several techniques.

MEDITATION

Meditation is an integral part of life in Asian cultures, whence it sprang and where it is tied up with the view of the world and with spiritualism. Western science has shown that meditation has deep and measurable relaxing effects which are inherently pleasant and useful. Although here Transcendental Meditation (TM) has gotten the most publicity, there are many schools of meditation. So whether or not you revere a maharishi for spiritual reasons, or for his business acumen, you may be able to turn to some type of meditation to your advantage.

All schools of meditation aim to focus your attention inward by concentrating on (meditating upon) the steady rhythm of your breathing, or on a single object, thought, word, or sound such as the mantra "om." By focusing your concentration so intently, your mind becomes empty of all distracting thoughts.

DEEP BREATHING

This is a simple technique that you can do on your own, after checking with your doctor. It actually relaxes your muscles and can slow down your heartbeat, lower your blood pressure, and increase blood flow to your hands and feet. Sitting or lying in a comfortable position, close your eyes, and try to empty your mind of all thoughts. Place your hand over your abdomen, inhale through the nose, slowly, to the count of four, while puffing up your stomach and letting your diaphragm expand and the air travel up to the chest, back, and shoulders, and imagining it filling your entire body. When you feel as full of air as you can be, hold it a second. Then slowly to the count of four, exhale through the mouth and feel the tension drain out of you along with the air. Repeat this, gradually slowing down the inhalation and exhalation to a count of ten and holding it for ten.

PROGRESSIVE RELAXATION
(Muscle Tensing and Relaxing)

This technique has been around since the 1930s, when Dr. Edmund Jacobson, a psychophysiologist, developed it. Since then, many variations have evolved, but they are all basically a way of systematically relaxing the body by alternately tensing and relaxing individual parts of it. It is easier to relax something that has been made very tense first: Using the principle of extremes, you first get to know how it feels to be really tense; then let go completely and thus get to know how it feels to be really relaxed. Here is an abbreviated form of progressive muscle relaxation which you might want to try.

In quiet surroundings, lie or sit down (lying is best) in a comfortable position, wearing comfortable, loosened clothing. Close your eyes and become aware of your body and your breath. You should breathe deeply, easily, and rhythmically throughout the exercise. Focus on your right foot and flex your toes back really hard; hold it this way for a few seconds, and then let it go completely limp and relaxed. Work up your right leg by tensing each muscle group and then letting it go completely, and making note of and enjoying the difference between the two sensations. Then do your left foot and leg. Then the hips, waist, back, chest, hands and arms, shoulders, neck, and scalp. Move to your face, open your mouth wide, raise your eyebrows, stare with wide open eyes. Next, scrunch your face and purse your lips as if you had just tasted something sour— and then completely relax those muscles. Stretch your arms overhead, point your toes, and stretch and tense every single muscle in your body at one time. Then relax. Return your focus to your breathing, and gradually open your eyes, and bring your awareness back to your surroundings.

HYPNOSIS AND SELF-HYPNOSIS

Sleeping and daydreaming are two altered states of consciousness; we enter these naturally and frequently. Hypnosis is thought to be an altered state too—one that has been used in some form for many years. Lately, it has been increasingly used by the medical and related professions for a number of reasons, often to relax patients before anxiety-producing procedures as drugless anesthesia, and as a means of controlling acute and chronic pain and discomfort.

Matthew Loscalzo, who lectures and trains others in hypnosis, feels that though "this technique is becoming increasingly utilized, a lot of people still have a lot of ignorance and misconceptions about hypnosis. People fear that the hypnotist has power over the patient, rather than it being an extension of some everyday normal processes, such as daydreaming or fantasy. Even in the deepest trances the patient is never really gone.'"

A hypnotist helps us enter the trance and may then go on to train us in self-hypnosis so we are no longer so dependent upon the skills and time of another person. The hypnotic state has been compared to a meditative trance—both are valuable sources of relaxation and lead to a sense of well-being. But hypnosis is more than entering a relaxed state—it is a goal-oriented technique used to focus on specific problems that are usually stress-related. It is generally agreed that when a person is in a deeply relaxed state, he or she is more open to "suggestion"—the introduction of a believable idea, thought, or image into a person's mind. As Mr. Loscalzo continues:

"Hypnosis is somewhat like a meditation technique. If people already know how to meditate, my work is half done. I ask them to put themselves into a meditative trance and we do the work in that state. But a trance itself doesn't do the work. It does nothing but put you in a relaxed state, which creates a medium for communication. Being in a relaxed state is not necessarily therapeutic in itself. It's a technique or a tool, or a way of thinking about treatment, it's not therapy."

Hypnosis and related techniques such as relaxation and desensitization help some patients cope with some of the side effects of chemotherapy and with some of the medical procedures that usually go along with it. Hypnosis can counteract conditioned aversions (such as anticipatory vomiting, which occurs before a chemotherapy treatment); post-treatment nausea and vomiting; phobic reactions (such as fear of a hypodermic or intravenous needle); acute or chronic anxiety (such as that surrounding a treatment or procedure, or surrounding the diagnosis of cancer); and some types of acute and chronic pain. It can also be used to relieve depression by overcoming the "learned helplessness" common to many patients and imparting a generalized sense of self-control.

VISUALIZING/CREATIVE IMAGING

Various forms of visualization have been used for many years in conjunction with hypnosis and relaxation to treat many ailments, complaints, and undesirable habits—pain, fears, overeating, and smoking. During visualization, people first enter a deeply relaxed state, and then create a mental picture of a desired goal or outcome. Overweight people, for example, picture themselves as thin. When cancer patients use visualization, they often imagine their cancer cells as weak and confused, their treatment and white blood cells are seen destroying the cancer cells, and their bodies are visualized as recovering and being healthy.

The use of visualization for cancer patients has become popular largely as the result of the pioneering work of Carl O. Simonton, a radiation oncologist, and his wife, Stephanie Matthew-Simonton, a psychologist. Together they established the Cancer Counseling and Research Center in Forth Worth, Texas, and then wrote a book, *Getting Well Again: A Step-by-Step Guide to Overcoming Cancer*, about their results. In it they state:

"It is our central premise that an illness is not purely a physical problem but rather a problem of the whole person, that it includes not only body but mind and emotions. We believe that emotional and mental states play a significant role both in *susceptibility* to disease, including cancer, and in *recovery* from all disease. We believe that cancer is often an indication of problems elsewhere in an individual's life, problems aggravated or compounded by a series of stresses six to eighteen months prior to onset of cancer. The cancer patient has typically responded to these problems and stresses with a deep sense of hopelessness, or 'giving up.' This emotional response, we believe, in turn triggers a set of physiological responses that suppress the body's natural defenses and make it susceptible to producing abnormal cells."

Their theories grew out of studies about stress published in the medical literature and from their own experiences and observations. Lawrence LeShan's work on the so-called cancer personality was particularly influential. In his book *You Can Fight for Your Life: Emotional Factors in the Causation of Cancer*, which was the result of twenty years' work with 500 cancer patients, this psychologist suggests that there is a general type of personality and emotional history common to cancer patients. He said this pattern prevailed in 76 percent of all the cancer patients he studied; but in only 10 percent of the non-cancer patient controls. This personality is characterized by feelings of helplessness and hopelessness and an all-or-none perspective with little room for compromise; this psychological orientation "Increases the chances of getting cancer and makes it more difficult for many individuals to fight for their lives when they do develop a malignancy."

The Simontons's conclusions became the cornerstone for their holistic program of cancer treatment (which included visualization, counseling, nutrition, and exercise), which their patients followed while being treated by their primary oncologist. According to the Simontons, their cancer patients at the Cancer Center in Texas—each of whom had a diagnosis of medically incurable cancer—lived on the average twice as long as patients who received medical treatment alone. And 51 percent of their patients maintained the same level of activity they had prior to the diagnosis, a sign that their quality of life was also higher than expected.

Medical doctors, nurses, psychiatrists, psychologists, and social workers use visualization, usually after other relaxation techniques have been firmly established with their patients. M. L. Frohling, for instance, begins first with an education component. She explains to patients that chemotherapy is a stressful situation and helps them understand the way they are perceiving and reacting physically to the treatment. She uses biofeedback to measure the physical effects and point them out to the patient. Then she teaches them breathing and progressive relaxation which they practice at home three times a day. "Once I see a patient is doing a lot of home practice and can really relax the body, I add visualization." She then uses visualization three ways:

> "I use it for rehearsal. The patients envision themselves getting the therapy, it coming into their bodies and killing the cancer cells. I have them picture themselves going through the treatment, feeling good, calm, relaxed, and in control. They feel themselves participating in their treatment process, seeing themselves healthy. We can start this a few days before the therapy is administered and then do it during the chemotherapy treatment itself, actually visualizing the drugs killing the confused cancer cells.
>
> "I also use it for manipulation, for pain reduction. I teach them how to manipulate pain by using some kind of symbol. For instance, they may assign a color and shape to areas of the body that are feeling pain; then the pain-free parts are assigned a light blue soothing color that gradually creeps into the colors where they feel the pain, slowly shrinking and easing the pain.
>
> "Finally, I use visualization as a mini-vacation. They visualize a safe, comfortable place that they enjoy going to and can relax in. Taking a vacation away from where you're at will create a relaxation response."

One patient describes her experiences with these techniques that she became interested in because of her anxiety and nausea:

> "I felt kind of silly at first. It's a crazy thing to imagine your own cancer cells and create your own Army of white cells to fight them. But believe it or not, you *are* able to visualize these things. As we get older, maybe we're stupid not to do things that are silly. Maybe we become too realistic.

"The self-hypnosis helped me stop the anticipatory anxiety and vomiting; it also eliminated the metallic taste in my mouth from the drugs. The doctor tried to help me control the nausea after the chemotherapy, but that he couldn't do. I think that's because I didn't believe in it as much as I should have.

"I think the thing with this is it gives you a sense of control of yourself. It's like your own personal chemo-therapy. It's something you can do for yourself. I think it is also a way of letting out hostilities. It takes me twenty-five minutes every day and it's hard to find the time to do it, but it's very relaxing and I feel such a sense of well-being. Even though I'm off chemo now, I'm continuing to do it."

Some proponents of visualization believe that the mind can actually control the cancer. There is no real proof of this in the form of the controlled studies that scientists have been trained to go by; there are only anecdotal material and uncontrolled studies. While the thought that we have the power within us to control our own minds and bodies to such an extent as to influence the course of our illness is an exhilarating one, it can also be frightening in its implications.

Critics of this view say it implies that we somehow caused the disease in the first place. As Susan Sontag writes in *Illness as Metaphor*, it manages to "put the onus of the disease on the patient." This is "preposterous" she says; it is a punishment, a moralistic view of the disease. It seems to me that once you become sold on the idea that you have caused and can therefore "uncause" your cancer, you become solely responsible for your disease. Under these conditions, it may be more devastating when there is a setback. If the cancer is not controlled, it follows that *you* alone are guilty of failure, or weakness, of a lack of faith, of wanting to die no matter how much you really want to live—a tremendously unfair additional burden for a cancer patient to have to bear.

Matthew Loscalzo says, "I do visualization and all that stuff. The literature shows that white blood cell counts can be raised through these techniques, and I'm comfortable with that. But I'm very skeptical of people who take people's money and say they are curing cancer."

Of the many therapists who are trained in the Simonton techniques, or closely related ones, few would go so far as to say that visualization alone can control cancer. Most use it in conjunction with other therapies, including conventional therapies such as chemotherapy, because it helps their patients feel more in control over their lives, and because it helps them tolerate the therapy better and come to have faith in it as a friend, not an enemy.

The Simontons say about this: "We all participate in our own health through our beliefs, our feelings, and our attitudes toward life, as well as in more direct ways such as through exercise and diet. In addition, our response to medical treatment is influenced by our beliefs about the effectiveness of the treatment and by the confidence we have in the medical team."

OTHER THERAPIES

There are many other therapies, disciplines, and practices that cancer patients have found help them cope with the mental and physical stresses of chemotherapy. Body work such as yoga, exercise, and massage therapies are one type. Expressive therapies such as dance therapy and art therapy are another—these enable people to be expressive in nonverbal ways. "People can be inhibited verbally—then can't talk about what's going on inside them," says M. L. Frohling. "But they can feel it. They might be able to move or draw and express it that way. When they do express it in some form, there is a sense of completeness and relaxation."

Laughter therapy is a new addition to the menu of stress-reducing techniques. The idea may make you laugh, but laughter is one of the best coping mechanisms there is. Norman Cousins put laughter therapy on the map with his well-known book, *Anatomy of an Illness*, which chronicles his use of humorous books, old episodes of "Candid Camera," and old Marx Brothers' movies to help him recover from a crippling degenerative disease.

There's nothing funny about having cancer, but we can still laugh at the world. Sometimes we can even laugh at ourselves—or appreciate the absurdities involved with our disease and our treatment. It's hard to imagine laughing when you've been throwing up for three hours straight, and you know you'll be doing the same thing every two weeks for the next year; when you're so weak you can barely drag yourself out of bed; when you're so pale and bald that even *you* don't want to be seen with you. And yet patients do find it within themselves to laugh. These things are so awful that people need to laugh—as an escape, a defense, and as a release of tension. Patients often joke about looking like Kojak, or majoring in Advanced Toilet Bowl, or how they might get arrested because their arms look like a junkie's. As one patient says, "It doesn't seem so awful when you laugh about it."

Your oncologist's attitude can encourage or discourage a healthy sense of humor about your situation. I sometimes spent more time joking and laughing than being treated. My doctor said I had the same type of humor you usually find in an oncologist. Dr. Charles Vogel of the comprehensive Cancer Center for the state of Florida likens the atmosphere on some oncology services to that of the M*A*S*H unit of film and TV fame. Los Angeles oncologist Dr. Michael Van Scoy-Mosher is a firm believer in the value of laughter for his patients:

"I think humor can be used—not that this isn't serious—but I found there's a real place for seeing it in an almost absurdist way. This view can be very useful. I remember, for example, I was treating a guy with a real sickening therapy for Hodgkin's disease. He happened to see me one day out in a store. The moment he saw me and his eyes met mine, he threw up. We both understood, but of course, nobody else in the store understood—they just saw this weird guy come in, throw up and leave. We had a good laugh about it later."

Scientists actually have an explanation as to why laughter does us so much good. When you laugh, many parts of your body contract—your chest, abdominal muscles, diaphragm, and lungs. Your systolic blood pressure soars, your pulse rate can double, adrenaline is pumped into your blood, and endorphin (the body's natural painkiller) may be released. A good belly laugh is like a mini-workout, an internal jogging. Afterward, everything goes back to normal or slightly below, which results in a release of tension and an all-round feeling of well-being.

For cancer patients in St. Joseph's Hospital in Houston, Texas, oncologist John S. Stehlin designed a "Living Room" based on the doctor's observations that patients who had positive attitudes and displayed moods of happiness and cheerfulness tended to get better results from treatment than those who were down. The upbeat activities offered include a library of comedy videotapes and regular joke-telling sessions. Some physicians are beginning to prescribe laughter therapy as a part of their overall treatment plans and are finding both physical and physiological health improvements. There are even official laugh therapists, such as Annette Goodman who treats cancer patients and who says that laughter is a cathartic process. "Once you laugh, you're no longer miserable. It brings people together."

Music can be quite therapeutic, too, and is being offered as an option to cancer patients at a growing number of medical facilities all over the country. Soothing classical and/or harp music is often used in conjunction with the relaxation techniques described earlier to make chemotherapy treatments more bearable, to help patients sleep, or to ease anxiety in general. A lung cancer patient who discovered music early during the course of her very difficult therapy said using her small cassette player and earphones during and after each treatment got her over the roughest spots.

Music has indeed been shown to have direct effects on the mind and body, although we're not yet sure exactly how. Music can generate feelings of serenity and relaxation, or cheerfulness and excitement, or gloom and melancholy; it can conjure up all sorts of mental images; it can affect our blood volume, our heart rate, and our blood pressure. Because it can affect us so powerfully, choose your playlist carefully. You may want to follow the advice of most music therapists who recommend that people with medical problems work with professionals who will teach you how to use music specifically to reduce yor perception of discomfort and create a positive state of mind.

CHAPTER 8

Diet and Nutrition

While good nutrition is important for everyone, no one really knows *exactly* what good nutrition is for the average healthy human being, let alone what is needed by the chemotherapy patient. Two facts have emerged from recent research, however. First of all: Diet and nutrition are an important source of support for those who are living under the special conditions and stresses that cancer and chemotherapy impose. And second: Nutrition is probably comprised to some degree in every person who undergoes chemotherapy.

HOW YOUR DIET AND NUTRITIONAL STATUS ARE AFFECTED

The chemicals used in cancer chemotherapy affect your mind and body and thus your diet in many ways. They cause a loss of appetite, a change in your ability to taste foods, nausea and vomiting, and changes in the mucosal lining of the mouth, esophagus, stomach, and intestines. All this can lead to alterations in the kinds and amounts of food you eat as well as your body's ability to absorb and utilize what you do eat. Some drugs can themselves chemically deplete or destroy nutrients in the body. As a result, chemotherapy alone can cause multiple obvious and not so obvious nutritional deficiencies.

In addition, the cancer patient is exposed to many other factors and conditions that deplete the body's supply of nutrients and/or increase its demand for them. Physical and psychological stress such as the diagnosis of cancer itself, surgery, and radiation have well-documented deleterious effects on nutritional status. The mere fact of being hospitalized—the physical and psychological stress of the treatments and the poor diet— has been shown to cause nutritional deficiencies. Other deficiencies or imbalances might be present due to the cancer itself, or as carry-overs from dietary conditions that contributed to the development of cancer in the first place.

My oncologist says:

> "It's well understood now that many patients who have gone through surgical operations and who are in the process of receiving toxic medications have serious nutritional deficiencies. One of the most serious forms of malnourishment that occurs anywhere on earth occurs in the modern hospital. A person is thought to be okay because he is on intravenous feeding. The fact of the matter is that the total amount of nutrition he receives over the course of twenty-four hours is about the same as a couple of Coca-Colas."

Consequently, chemotherapy patients often lose weight (although some actually gain it), become deficient in many vitamins and minerals, lose energy, and generally fall into a malnourished, unhealthy state at the very time they need to remain as strong and healthy as possible to fight the cancer, repair the damage done by the disease, and withstand the side effects of therapy. This not only lessens their quality of life while on chemotherapy, but it could be setting them up for problems in the future.

WHERE TO GET HELP

The ways that nutrition, diet cancer, and chemotherapy interrelate is a frustratingly complicated field of study. Much more work needs to be done. Yet evidence is accumulating and you can put it to work for your benefit. As D. M. Hegsted, professor of nutrition at the Harvard School of Public Health declares in "Optimal Nutrition," an article published in the May 1979 supplement of *Cancer*: "The fact that we do not know the optimal solution cannot and does not prevent us from using whatever relevant evidence is available to make the best judgment possible. If we wait until we know everything we need to know, we will wait forever." He is addressing the problem of nutritional links with the onset of cancer, but the same arguments are being made for treatment too.

Self-education is the first step toward making that judgment. What follows is a brief outline of the various types of thinking on the subject. Some suggestions are very well-founded and accepted; you can safely adopt many of them on your own. But findings are often contradictory or inconclusive, making some principles and theories less sound, and perhaps less safe than others. Because the issue is so complex and important, only a qualified dietician, nutritionist, or nutrition-oriented physician can intelligently advise you about making any drastic changes in your diet or taking large doses of vitamins, minerals, or other nutritional supplements. Although you should let your oncologist know if you are concerned about nutrition, you shouldn't expect your oncologist to dispense nutritional advice—most traditional doctors are lamentably ignorant about nutrition; some are consequently downright hostile toward the nutritional approach to anything.

This problem is well-recognized by experts in the nutrition field, be they of a conservative or progressive bent. However, this state of affairs is gradually improving; imagine my own surprise when my surgeon, who had always seemed very traditionally minded, recently started asking me whether I take vitamins B, C, E, and selenium! Lisa Logan, nutrition support clinical dietician at Presbyterian Denver Hospital says:

"Many oncology patients have very complex medical problems and frequently nutrition may be the last problem addressed. The current literature, which supports early nutrition intervention to lessen complications and improve tolerance to therapy, can no longer be ignored. So I have seen a gradual improvement in the awareness of physicians I work with. Also, many hospital outpatient clinics have nutritionists that deal specifically with oncology patients. Physicians concerned with the importance of nutrition will refer their patients for more extensive nutrition assessment and intervention."

Shari Lieberman, a nutritionist and registered dietician in private practice, speaks from her own experience:

"The problem with conventional doctors is not that they don't believe in nutrition, but that they are uneducated in that area. They don't admit this to their patients, but they admit it to me. They tell me to do what I think is best, and to let them know what I'm doing. The added need for nutrients during chemotherapy is well documented, particularly as it relates to physical and physiological stress. So doctors that argue about this are just not reading. Maybe there's a little bit of tunnel vision.

"Although there are some hospital dieticians who are doing progressive work, generally they are conservative. A nutritionist found through a health food store, on the other hand, is obviously working with supplements and not just the four food groups. Try to get the names of a couple of them; then ask where they got their educations and what they got their degrees in. Are they registered dieticians? People call themselves nutritionists who are not, and nutritionists need a background in biochemistry to understand the subtleties of nutrition and make intelligent decisions about the published findings."

Dr. Michael Schachter of the Mountainview Medical Associates, a private practice holistic center, thinks oncologists tend to resist the idea of nutritional therapy as an adjunct to chemotherapy for several reasons:

"In some respects the two approaches are antagonistic—one tends to break down the body, the other tends to build it up. Or it may be related to the old expression, 'If you're not up on something, you're down on it.' They may think if there's some value to nutrition then they should be doing it too—but they're not doing it. So to protect themselves they have a very strong negative feeling about it.

"The position of many oncologists is they say the

nutritional approach has not been sufficiently proven. But studies relating nutritional factors to cancer may take many years to complete and cancer patients can't wait for these to be finished before taking action to help themselves. Some chemotherapy patients feel pretty terrible and clinically they feel a lot better when they undertake a nutritionally supportive program along with their chemotherapy.

"We are happy to work with oncologists, if they are willing to work with us. Frequently oncologists do not support their patients being on a nutritional program, but patients are convinced that it will help. Consequently, patients surreptitiously undertake nutritional programs. We often get feedback from the patient that his oncologist is extremely pleased at how well he is doing; that the patient is zipping through the therapy with a minimum of side effects. I can also say that more and more oncologists, though skeptical of nutritional therapeutic approaches doing much good, are not taking as hard a line as they did previously. They say to go ahead and do if you want to, as long as you take the chemotherapy too."

My oncologist, who stresses the importance of individualizing all aspects of cancer treatment, sometimes suggests adding nutritional therapy to the chemotherapy regimen, despite its "unproven" nature.

"My approach is that there are many things we don't know in medicine. But there are substances which are of use in assisting people to be able to perform better and do better which have negligible side effects. These can be useful in improving the strength of a person who is receiving therapy for malignancy. So I have tried to bring in elements that might be of benefit in terms of improving the body's strength. I have had to look at many sources, both traditional and nontraditional. Traditional approaches tend to look at data more critically and use double-blind testing to validate the doses of substances that are required. The nontraditional ones tend to say, 'Why don't we just try this and see what happens.' That latter approach has also produced some interesting effects. So I am in the position at this point in time of having to take somewhat sketchy, experimental data and apply it, perhaps in advance of its complete understanding.

"My basic point of view is that you keep your eyes open. You keep trying to apply as many things that may help as you can get your hands on, without being kooky. One has to be modest but listen to everything. I feel that as an internist I have to be well-versed in everything that happens."

WHAT GOOD NUTRITION CAN DO FOR YOU

Proper nutrition can help you four important ways.

IMPROVES TOLERANCE OF THERAPY

A well-nourished body is stronger and more resilient than a poorly nourished one. Studies have shown that nutrition can decrease the severity and duration of side effects such as vomiting, nausea, weakness, lowered immunity, and susceptibility to infection. There may be other special side effects that we do not know about yet, but in general people who eat well while on chemotherapy tend to feel better, and stay more physically active and more alert mentally.

INCREASES THE EFFECTIVENESS OF THERAPY

When you feed yourself, you also feed your cancer cells. Studies have shown that well-fed cancer cells multiply more readily and so are more susceptible to anticancer drugs than are slow growing, undernourished cells. In addition, a good nutritional status may allow you to withstand higher doses of drugs and so increase the effectiveness of the therapy in that way as well.

SPEEDS RECOVERY FROM TREATMENTS

Nutrients are the building blocks your body uses to rebuild the normal tissues that have been affected by the chemotherapy. If the proper nutrients in the proper amounts are available, the recovery process takes place much more quickly and efficiently than when deficiencies are present.

REGULATES YOUR WEIGHT

Many people lose weight on chemotherapy but some (notably women on chemotherapy for breast cancer) gain weight. Underweight and overweight are both undesirable for the chemotherapy patient: They can lead to weakness, lethargy, depression, embarrassment, and lack of self-esteem. Being careful about what you eat will help control both these extremes.

THE BASIC FOUR + ONE

All approaches to nutritional support for the chemotherapy patient are grounded in the concept of a well-balanced diet. Simply stated, a balanced diet contains a variety of foods that will give you the vitamins, minerals, protein, carbohydrates, fats, and water needed to keep your body working normally. In order to help people get the variety of foods in the right amounts, the basic four food groups were established. Adhering to this basic plan is good practice for everyone, chemotherapy patients included. Since some anticancer drugs can affect the bladder or kidneys, it is important for you to include a fifth group: liquids (water, juices, tea, broth, soup). Everyday's menu should include:

Fruit and vegetables: four servings (two of each)
Meat, fish, poultry, eggs, cheese: three servings
Grains: four servings
Milk and milk products: two servings
Liquids: eight to twelve glasses.

Even though you may not be feeling well, or don't feel like eating these particular foods, it is important to eat well. If side effects make it difficult for you to eat according to this plan or if you have lost or are losing weight, turn to the chapter on gastrointestinal side effects for tips on overcoming your difficulties. For instance, you might need to add extra protein and calories, which are required after surgery to help you heal and during chemotherapy to help your body replace lost cells. Some patients are advised to add liquid nutritional supplements to their diets. Generally, a multivitamin/mineral supplement, which will help make up for the nutrients that your diet is lacking, can be taken safely and is advised. In *A Comprehensive Guide for Cancer Patients and Their Families*, Dr. Ernest Rosenbaum writes:

> "In some cases vitamin and mineral supplements may be needed because of the side effects of certain types of cancer or of therapy, which may result in vitamin or mineral losses or increased requirements. Vitamin and mineral supplements may also be needed by patients who are unable to eat a balanced diet, or who have loss of appetite, malabsorption or weight loss, or who drink or smoke excessively."

The majority of chemotherapy patients fit into at least one of these categories. Remember, too, not to rely solely on supplements—real foods contain nutritional elements that supplements don't, perhaps some we don't even know exist. (In extreme cases of advanced cancer of severe weight loss, an oncologist or dietician may put patients on supplemental tube feedings—either through tubes inserted into the stomach or small intestine or through intravenous feedings.)

THE NEW GUIDELINES: IMPROVING UPON THE BASIC FOUR

The advantage of the basic four food groups model is that it is fairly easy for the average person to follow: The typical American diet can easily satisfy its requirements so no major changes are needed in the way we're used to eating. This is in some ways a disadvantage because it has been discovered that as a population we are not eating as well as we thought we were, and we should make changes. It's possible to appear to be following the basic four and still get too little of some nutrients and too much of others. For example, you may not accept the concept of catsup as a vegetable but readily accept canned string beans or french fries, which are also fairly low in the hierarchy of wholesome food.

There is so much evidence that the typical American diet is a contributing factor to many diseases—cancer being one of them—that even conservative government agencies (such as the Department of Agriculture, the National Cancer Institute, the Senate Select Committee of Nutrition and Human Needs, the Health, Education, and Welfare Department, and the National Academy of Sciences) have released very similar dietary guidelines urging Americans to change their eating habits. The National Academy of Sciences surveyed the scientific literature and concluded that cancers of most major sites are influenced by dietary patterns. Based on animal studies and observation of many human populations, it has found that we eat too much salt, too much fat, too much sugar, too much cholesterol, and too much food in general. And our health is suffering because of our indulgence. If you want to take further steps to safeguard your health, use these guidelines when choosing from the basic four food groups.

Several studies show that people who consume greater quantities of fat have a higher incidence of cancers of the breast, bowel, and prostate. Americans should reduce the current level of their fat intake by more than one fourth, so it accounts for 30 percent or less of their total calories rather than the usual 40 percent. Dietary fat should consist of equal proportions of saturated, monounsaturated, and polyunsaturated fat. To do this, we should eat less beef and other fatty meats, reduce our consumption of cheese and other whole-milk, full-fat dairy products, and avoid fried foods.

VEGETABLES, FRUITS, AND WHOLE GRAINS

These foods are high in vitamin C and in beta-carotene, which is converted to vitamin A in the body. There is evidence that shows that these nutrients protect against the development of cancer. Oranges, grapefruit, apricots, cantaloupes, peaches, strawberries, dark leafy green vegetables, carrots, winter squash, tomatoes, green peppers, and sweet potatoes—all are high in one or both of vitamins A and C. Cruciferous vegetables (broccoli, brussels sprouts, cabbage, and cauliflower) contain these vitamins plus certain compounds that research indicates can increase the body's capacity to convert carcinogens into harmless substances. These foods are also high in fiber, as are whole grains such as whole wheat bread and bran cereal. Lower fiber consumption has been implicated in bowel and breast cancer, and the National Cancer Institute recommends that we increase our intake. It has been suggested that about half our total calories be derived from these complex carbohydrates and naturally occurring sugars, and that our intake of refined and processed carbohydrates be reduced to 10 percent.

SMOKED OR CURED FOODS

Pickled, smoked, and salt-cured foods appear to increase the incidence of cancers of the stomach and esophagus. Japan, Iceland, and China, where these foods are consumed in great quantities, have higher incidences of these cancers. So avoid consuming a lot of hot dogs, bologna, salami and sausages, ham, bacon, and smoked fish; salt should be reduced to five grams per day.

ALCOHOL

Alcohol, especially when combined with cigarette smoking, has been connected with higher rates of cancer of the mouth, larynx, liver, and lungs. Drinking "in moderation" is advised—probably no more than two drinks per day.

ADDED BENEFITS FROM NUTRITIONAL THERAPY

Although these guidelines are a step in the right direction, there are many experts who say they do not go far enough—not for the average population and especially not for the cancer patient who is at high-risk for disease already and who is being further weakened by various therapies.

They point out that first of all, since cancer chemotherapy patients are at a high risk to develop second cancers and other illnesses, they should modify their diets as much as possible to reduce this risk. They feel that the recommended daily allowances (RDAs) of vitamins and minerals in the so-called balanced diet are hard for anyone—and impossible for the chemotherapy patient—to get every day. They also claim that these RDAs are far too low anyway for optimum health in the average person and do not even begin to answer the needs of the chemotherapy patient. They argue that large doses of vitamins and minerals should be added to the nutritional regimen because they can protect organs from the toxicity of the drugs, counteract the carcinogenic activity of the drugs and other chemicals in the food and the environment, and improve the functioning of the immune system—which plays a role in destroying cancer cells but is being weakened by the therapy.

My oncologist says he is "not a megavitamin person" and thinks it's important to distinguish between megadoses of vitamins and large doses of vitamins. He will sometimes prescribe "large reasonable" doses of vitamins and minerals that might be useful as adjunctives in terms of trying to build the body.

> "Data produced by the National Cancer Institute, for example, have shown that vitamin E is useful as an antioxidant, and it has many other remarkable effects and no negative ones. There's lots of evidence to suggest that zinc is useful in the management of immunodeficiency disease of many origins. There is some data to suggest that selenium is useful under some circumstances. In reasonable doses, vitamin C does tend to promote restoration of normal tissue strength. Vitamin A in reasonable doses has been shown to be an immuno-stimulant under some circumstances. B vitamins have been shown to be useful during the recovery from many conditions; B vitamins are rapidly used up during cell death and cell restoration. So, for instance, one or two milligrams of vitamin B_1 just isn't enough."

In Dr. Schachter's holistic practice, nutrition is a cornerstone:

> "Patients must have appropriate quantities of each of the nutrients in order to optimally support their body defenses. At the same time, nontherapeutic toxic substances

should be eliminated as much as possible. We start out by recommending the elimination of junk foods, refined carbohydrates, chemicals, and so on. We emphasize the ingestion of complex carbohydrates—whole grains, vegetables, nuts, and seeds—and that patients try to cut down on their meat, and get organic beef if they can. And then we add a nutritional supplementation program—vitamins, minerals, enzymes—as a kind of insurance.

"With regard to cancer, we're especially interested in trying to stimulate the body's defense system. We believe in the surveillance theory that people are developing cancer cells all the time. So we try to supplement liberally with nutrients that are thought to improve the body's defense system. We're also interested in protecting the organs against chemotherapy. One of the things that chemotherapeutic agents can do is form free radicals which damage the cell membranes and lead to carcinogenesis. By taking large (but not toxic) doses of vitamins A, C, and E, and selenium, you're nourishing the organs that are being bombarded by toxic substances and protecting them from some of the damage."

Shari Lieberman comments:

"I'm not against chemotherapy per se. It's just that it's done in a very non-thinking way. It's done to people who aren't eating, who aren't taking any supplements, who end up with multiple nutritional deficiencies, which is the last thing you want to do to a cancer patient.

"When people talk about eating a well-balanced, nutritional diet and they say you can get everything you need from food, that is uneducated. In order to get the RDAs of all the nutrients—which as far as I'm concerned are the bare minimum—you have to eat about 2,500 calories a day. That's a lot for the average person, and for people on chemotherapy—forget it.

"The thing that I emphasize for people who are going to take chemotherapy is that they can use nutrition to minimize the risks and negative effects of the chemotherapy. You can take supplements of selenium and vitamin E, which are antioxidants, and of A or betacarotene."

Progressive nutritional therapy for the chemotherapy patient seeks to improve his or her health generally and protect specifically against carcinogens (such as anticancer drugs). It is based on three principles.

1. Avoid foods and nontherapeutic substances that are known to be or are highly suspected of being carcinogenic, or that make the body a hospitable place for cancer to develop.
2. Include nutrients that bolster the body's own defenses.
3. Include substances that have the direct or indirect ability to inhibit the formation of cancer in the body.

It sounds simple, but the practice is not without its controversies. We don't know everything about the way the body responds either to chemotherapy or to the various nutrients, let alone about how chemotherapy and nutrients interact in the body. What to take? How much to take? Large doses of zinc, for example, have been shown to inhibit tumor formation in animals—but under other experimental conditions zinc may actually enhance tumor growth. Other equally contradictory findings can be cited for many other nutrients.

For many years these concepts and claims have been lumped with the alternative therapies, and so dismissed as worthless in the treatment or prevention of cancer. However, aspects of them have recently begun to capture the interest of members of the medical establishment. Most of the evidence so far is based on epidemiological studies that correlate the life-styles of large segments of the population with cancer incidence, on animal studies, and on undocumented human experiments. The National Cancer Institute is testing the effects of vitamin A, beta-carotene, vitamins C and E, and selenium to see whether they have an impact on cancer risk. The evidence is steadily accumulating that they do, and the case for supplementation, especially for the cancer patient being treated with toxic drugs, is getting stronger every day.

In one intriguing study done at the University of Wisconsin, breast cancer patients with high blood levels of vitamin A responded twice as well to chemotherapy as did women with lower levels. Two theories are being advanced to explain the results: Vitamin A helps protect against toxicity of the drugs; and the vitamin actually interacts with the drug to increase its potency against cancer cells.

Before I began chemotherapy, my oncologist gave me a nutritional evaluation. Based on lab tests and dietary analysis, he suggested a few changes and added nutritional supplements. I took (and still take) doses much higher than the RDAs. Knowing I was doing something that was perhaps protecting me from some of the harmful effects of chemo helped put my mind at ease. It formed an integral part of my overall therapy and ability to tolerate the drugs psychologically and perhaps physically too. Oncologists say that women on adjuvant chemotherapy for breast cancer typically have minimal side effects as I did. But I also have met many women who were devastated by it. I have no way of knowing to which of these two groups I would have belonged and whether the handfuls of vitamin pills made any difference. But I think and hope they did; just as I took chemotherapy to help fight my cancer, my nutritional regimen meant I wasn't going to take chemo lying down. It made me feel more confident and secure, and less afraid of the therapy and what it was doing to the rest of me while it killed the cancer cells.

CHAPTER 9

Exercise

While many oncologists advise their patients to stay active and try to live a life as normal as possible, few recommend an exercise program as a specific support therapy for those on chemotherapy. It is mentioned only in passing in books about the treatment of cancer, with the Simontons' *Getting Well Again* and the Rosenbaums' *A Comprehensive Guide for Cancer Patients and Their Families* being the two notable exceptions. This is surprising, since most of us by now know about at least some of the benefits we can derive from exercise. Regular exercise can play an important role in overall health, in our body image, body awareness, self-esteem, and self-sufficiency. It strengthens us and keeps us limber. It is a superb outlet for stress and tension, and a proven nondrug antidote to the blues and the blahs.

There are basically two reasons that chemotherapy patients are not advised to exercise: Physicians either are under the impression that it is of no benefit or believe that chemotherapy patients are too weak and frail to exercise. Generally, neither of these is true.

Linda E. Perkin, a registered physical therapist and exercise physiologist, is the former coordinator of the Oncology Fitness Program at Denver Presbyterian Medical Center. Ms. Perkin worked with cancer patients for six years at Presbyterian and

133

is now in private practice. She concedes that there are a few oncologists who are very progressive and do recommend that their chemotherapy patients exercise. Others, however, may think, "Oh don't bother them, just let them lie there. I think perhaps they focus so much on chemotherapy that they don't consider recommending generally healthy things like exercise."

In 1983 Ohio State University Comprehensive Cancer Center conducted a formal pilot project to study the physical and psychological effects of an exercise program on women with breast cancer. This was the first formal study of this nature ever done and was designed to compare a relatively aggressive rehabilitation program with the standard conservative approach. Dr. James Neidhart, the former deputy director of the cancer center, says: "This project met with a fair amount of resistance from physicians and lay people on our Human Use Committee. They felt that people with this type of cancer on these drugs should not be subjected to exercise, that the drugs are too toxic to allow it."

The study, which consisted of ten to twelve weeks of a combination of twenty minutes of aerobic training on a stationary bicycle plus stretching, demonstrated that some very positive results can be obtained by people receiving chemotherapy. Not only did the subjects not lose any of their fitness, they actually experienced an improvement of 20 percent. This was comparable to the control group of nonchemo subjects and may indicate that at least some chemo patients do not have to "just lie there." Maryl Winningham, exercise physiologist at Ohio State University and director of the study, cautions that it was a small pilot study. "It is important to realize that these are preliminary findings and it is dangerous to draw conclusions for all chemo patients." Nevertheless, she and others are very gratified by the result and she goes on, in following quote to give further evidence that the stereotype of the weak, sick cancer chemotherapy patient is not an inevitability. Dr. Winningham placed ads in *Runner's World, Nautilus Magazine*, and *Bicycling*, asking that cancer patients who exercised contact Ohio State. She tells of the replies:

"We got over two hundred and fifty responses—all ages, all types of cancers, all stages, from all over the country. These were people who said 'I am not going to sit down and die. I'm going to stay active as long as I can.' One

woman wrote us a letter about her husband who was a
runner. He ran on a Wednesday, entered the hospital on
the next Sunday, and died on that Monday. That is not
your typical picture of a cancer patient. You can carry
on the fight as long as you live."

Dr. William Grace, chief of oncology at New York's St.
Vincent's Hospital, feels:

"Patients with cancer tend to baby themselves and they
tend to get babied. It's good, I think, to emphasize that
they remain very active, to emphasize their health rather
than their illness. So we recommend a regular exercise
program for most patients. There are people who run in
races while on chemotherapy. Those high-performance
folks do terrifically. People who are physically active
seem to tolerate the chemotherapy. They tolerate more
drugs, they have fewer side effects, and they often have
a longer survival. Nobody knows why. It may be that
they got more poison—but they do better."

These days it is fairly likely that the cancer patient has been
on some kind of exercise program before the diagnosis and
treatment, and would like to continue afterward. Active people
want to remain as active as possible but may have questions
about whether they should continue, what form of exercise is
best, how much to do, will it hurt the action of the drugs or
deplete the body of the energy it needs to fight the cancer and
the side effects of chemotherapy. They—as well as people who
have not been particularly active—should be encouraged to
exercise because it has been found that many of the common
side effects of chemotherapy can be minimized in the intelligent
use of exercise.

THE BENEFIT OF EXERCISE

Exercise pays off in these specific ways for the chemotherapy patient.

INCREASE IN ENERGY

It is well known that rather than making you tired, exercise actually gives you more energy. Your muscles become stronger and more flexible; your body is able to do things with more ease and efficiency. With aerobic exercise especially, the heart and lungs get a workout. As a result, these systems are strengthened, the blood flow increases, as do the number of red blood cells which carry oxygen, and endurance improves. The more you do, the more you can do. Maryl Winningham says: "We think the right kind of exercise helps maintain energy levels. If a person feels tired and just sits around, the enzymes that make energy in the body start going down the toilet—literally. The more you lie around, the worse you feel, and the more you lie around. People are just waiting to feel better, and they don't. Unnecessary bed rest is a killer."

PSYCHOLOGICAL LIFT

Being physically capable and active is a positive step toward participating in your treatment and your life, especially if you have not been exercising much in the past. Regular exercise gives you a sense of vitality and physical accomplishment at the time you need it the most. It is well accepted that exercise can help you develop a clear, positive outlook.

Dr. Ward F. Cunningham-Rundles, an oncologist at Memorial Sloan-Kettering in New York, who encourages many of his cancer patients to exercise regularly, reasons:

"There's evidence to suggest that exercise tends to release endorphins and that tends to make one feel better for many elaborate reasons. I also suspect that when a person exercises it tends to increase the amount of circulation to every part of the body, thus encouraging the turnover of end products from the tissues, and that tends to make one feel better."

Endorphins, the morphinelike compounds released by the brain during workouts, produce a "high" and are the body's own painkillers. With endorphins coursing through your bloodstream, you feel a sense of well-being, possibly even euphoria. Exercise can also help reduce anxiety and stress, and it provides a direct physical outlet for whatever frustrations and hostilities you may feel.

"Exercise lets cancer patients feel that they are maintaining control," says Maryl Winningham, pointing out another plus for chemo patients, "and this is of course a critical thing." The increase or maintenance in the level of self-care, independence, and economic productivity provides a real lift. It has been found that depression, which is one of the most common emotional states in a cancer patient, is relieved by exercise. Some doctors routinely prescribe exercise for depressed patients.

As healthy, attractive changes take place in your body and mind, you realize that your physical limitations are not what you thought they were. In addition, even a few minutes of exercise can be like a short vacation that takes your mind off of cancer, chemotherapy, and how rotten you feel. One patient confesses:

> "I started jogging with a friend just after I stopped the chemo. I decided I had to do something to keep myself from feeling so blah. I just had no energy and we thought that maybe jogging would help. And it did. I enjoyed it. If you stop thinking about the worst, you can do things that you didn't think you could do before—your job, keeping up with the other person. Maybe if I used my muscles a little more I wouldn't have felt so blah while I was on the chemo."

And if you indulge in sports it is especially enjoyable—because of the company and because it's just plain fun.

I was a fitness nut before I got cancer, and I continued to exercise every chance I got. I wasn't up to running while on chemo, but I could swim and do calisthenics at home and at my gym. No one there except for one instructor knew I was on chemo. It was a great ego boost to see I could do just about everything that "normal" people could, and in many cases, even more. It made me feel less like a freak, less sorry for myself, and less that my life was a tragedy. I felt proud to be able to do as much as I did and relieved to be able to hold onto that part of the old me.

Physical exercise is an important symbol of health and vitality. If you have been exercising prior to your diagnosis and treatment, keeping physically active in an important affirmation of the continuity of your life and your life-style. In a time when so much may be changing, maintaining your exercise regimen as close to normal as possible assures you that your body—and your life—will go on and are not falling apart completely. If you can still swim laps, run around the park, dance, touch your toes, things don't seem quite so bad.

DECREASE IN NAUSEA AND VOMITING

"Exercise seems to cause a decrease in the nausea and vomiting that chemotherapy patients suffer," says Lin Perkin. She continues:

"We haven't been able to come up with anything scientifically definitive as to the physiological mechanism, but it may be due to the fact that hypermotility in the gastrointestinal tract tends to make people more nauseated. When you exercise, blood is diverted from the digestive system and into the muscles. Since there's less action in the gut and more somewhere else, this could be one of the mechanisms of decreased nausea. Or it may just be part of the proven psychological benefits of exercise—the fact of being active, not sitting around and brooding about the way you feel, or anticipating the way you're going to feel."

Dr. Winningham says that the patients in her study program felt less nauseated within about five minutes of exercising and maintained this for the rest of the day.

I was plagued by a constant low-level queasiness for most of my time on chemo. Exercise made it better, and swimming made it vanish completely.

STIMULATION OF THE IMMUNE SYSTEM

There is evidence that vigorous exercise stimulates the immune system, possibly in many ways. This is important for the chemotherapy patient whose immune system is regularly being compromised. Some of the effects may be due to the stress-reducing ability of exercise, but this is not well documented. However, studies have shown that endurance (aerobic) exercise increases the number of circulating white blood cells in the body.

"People who exercise—particularly aerobically—tend to keep their white cells up," says Lin Perkin. "The count still drops, but it stays within a safer range. Not that you produce anymore, but the turbulence of your blood brings them out of storage. So patients who have had a drop in their white count from chemotherapy can bring their immune systems back up by being active. This may help keep infections away and increase the effectiveness of chemotherapy by allowing the patient to accept a little more chemo, which might otherwise be held up or held back because of a low white blood cell count."

Although there is general agreement that exercise can have a beneficial effect on the immune system and the white cell count, there is conflicting evidence as to the particulars and some doubt as to the implications. Maryl Winningham, for instance, points out that there is a temporary rise in the white count during and immediately following intense exercise, and that patients probably should not exercise vigorously immediately before having a blood test. She cautions:

> "We are unsure about how chronic exercise affects the white cell count. Our hunch is that it might help stabilize it. Studies by the Russians demonstrate instability of the white count as a result of inactivity—the count fluctuates and the cells break down. We can't say categorically that it improves the count, but we do know that a lack of exercise seems to have a negative effect."

Dr. Cunningham-Rundles says he has "every reason to believe that patients who exercise do better," but that there's some question as to the amount and duration of the exercise and its beneficial effect on the immune system. He explains:

> "The situation is analogous to the relationship between alcohol and hypertension: A little bit will probably relax you a bit, but more will push your blood pressure up. In the same way, moderate exercise will likely improve immune function in many different ways. But if you've

ever taken care of marathoners, you'll find they get sick all the time. The stress they put on their bodies is tremendous. It's important to get some exercise, but beyond a certain point, it uses up important body-building blocks."

OTHER BENEFITS

Exercise has many other effects on the body that are of interest to the chemotherapy patient. It helps prevent osteoporosis (weakening of the bones) and coronary-artery disease. It stimulates the process of digestion, absorption, metabolism, and elimination, and so can help fight constipation.

It can help you sleep better on the one hand, and stimulate the brain on the other—endurance exercises may improve memory, mood, and attention span.

In addition, it is an invaluable tool for regulating weight. Many people lose weight while on chemotherapy; exercise can help you gain weight or prevent you from losing it because it can stimulate a waning appetite. Conversely, for people who gain weight from chemotherapy, activity helps prevent weight gain by burning up calories and raising your metabolism so calories are being burned even when you are not exercising. (Incidentally, Dr. Winningham comments on her study of women on chemotherapy for breast cancer, "The group as a whole did not gain any weight." And I didn't gain any weight either; although I got a little bloated tummy from the prednisone, I actually lost seven pounds during chemo.) Also, exercise gives you a sense of well-being and relieves boredom, which you might otherwise be tempted to alleviate through overeating.

WHAT, WHEN, AND HOW

No matter how weak and vulnerable you feel, you can do something that will in some way be beneficial. As the Simontons point out, cancer patients are capable of far more physical activity than most people usually assume. All that's needed sometimes is a little encouragement:

"Before the chemo I used to run up to six miles a day. But while on it I couldn't run for five minutes. My husband encouraged me to try other exercise—he's the type of person who pushes to the limit, and in a lot of respects that paid off for me. I'd say to him, 'What are you doing to me—I can't do this.' But I accomplished a lot more than I would have. He'd say, 'C'mon, you're going to go for a hike in the woods' or something like that. Physically I didn't feel any better after exercising, but psychologically I did."

Three days of bed rest can decrease a person's stamina by 25 percent. The longer you remain inactive, the harder it will be for you to regain strength. Even if you have been bedridden or inactive for some time, you should try to become as active as you were before the disease and its treatment took its effect.

When lying in a bed, you can wiggle your toes, raise your arms and legs, sit up, do head circles, shrug your shoulders, and inhale and exhale deeply. Try the deep-breathing or the muscle-tensing/relaxing exercises in Chapter 7. When you can't, get up and walk around, even if it's just around the room. These gentle forms of activity will help you restore and maintain your bodily functions, increase your body awareness, and relax you.

With your doctor's permission, you can begin some form of exercise soon after surgery and continue during chemotherapy. A surgeon might give you recuperative exercises that relate specifically to restoring bodily function after your surgery, or refer you to a physical therapist or a rehabilitation program, such as one of the ones offered to postmastectomy women at YMCAs, hospitals, and through the American Cancer Society's Reach to Recovery.

If you've been active, you will probably want to continue to resume your regular regimen in some form as soon as possible. But if you're new to exercise, if you've had surgery, or if you have stopped exercising for any reason, many of the guidelines you should follow resemble those applicable to anyone who starts exercising: Start slowly, build up gradually, begin each session with a light warm-up and end with a cooldown; stop when it hurts, slow down when you become too winded to speak. You'll be amazed at how much you can do, but if you notice irregular heartbeats, dizziness, nausea, chest pain, or difficulty breathing, stop and consult your doctor.

For some, ordinary activities such as walking, shopping,

cleaning, making the bed, climbing stairs, gardening, and playing with children might be enough. Others will want to continue or begin a more serious exercise program. There are many kinds of exercises that can improve your fitness level at all phases of your treatment, and dozens of books and classes. (It's wise for rookies to see a professional at first to get the proper technique.)

The Simontons suggest that you do whatever you like and whatever you can manage, but that you aim for one hour of exercise three times a week. This is the program prescribed to heart patients; anything less than that isn't as consistently beneficial. Jogging, alone or combined with walking, fast walking, bike riding, climbing stairs, and aerobic dancing are all recommended.

Swimming is also excellent, and many chemotherapy patients report that plunging into the water feels "great." You don't have to know how to swim to reap the benefits of the water's buoyance; water therapy is especially useful after surgery to avoid injury and during chemotherapy when your muscle strength is diminished. You can still perform movements in water that would be more difficult, and possibly injurious, on dry land. As soon as my surgeon gave me the go-ahead, I was back in the water. I began to do light water exercises and then swam a few laps. I eventually worked up to a mile and it felt better than it ever had before. The moment I dove into the water, the nausea disappeared, and so did the rest of the world. If it were possible, I would have stayed in the pool the whole nine months of treatment.

In his book *Do Not Go Gentle*, Herb Howe wrote that swimming in particular recharged him; "My pride in pulling against the water and rolling into a flip turn washed away any notions of defeat, dejection, and death." He remembered that Florence Chadwick, the marathon swimmer, had said, "Life in the water is less complicated."

Dr. William Grace says they often recommend the book, *Royal Canadian Air Force Exercise Plans for Physical Fitness*, at St. Vincent's because "The exercises start off at a very low level and build up gradually. They are also only twelve to fifteen minutes long," he points out, "and it's a very convenient way to judge progress or lack thereof. They're boring exercises, but they are good and they can be done without fancy equipment. A lot of people also walk or jog—and we recommend that."

The guidelines and precautions are pretty much the same as for noncancer patients, with a few exceptions. Maryl Winningham recommends that patients do not exercise for at least twenty-four hours after having a chemotherapy treatment. "At least nothing that will get their heart rates up. There is a possibility of diverting the chemicals into the muscle cells, which don't normally get a large blood flow, and away from the tumor cells."

Both Dr. Winningham and Ms. Perkin warn patients that if there are metastases to the bone, high-concussive types of exercises such as running and jumping are dangerous; they recommend activities that put a minimum amount of force (from the body's own weight) on the skeleton such as swimming, bicycling, and stretching. They also mention the need to modify the usual formula for obtaining the target heart rate during aerobic exercise in some cases. Ms. Perkin says if patients are very debilitated, she begins with the figure 220, the maximum human heart rate, from which she subtracts the age, then the resting heart rate. She then multiplies by 60 or 70 percent and finally reads the resting heart rate. In cardiotoxic therapies, she'll usually have patients use 60 to 50 percent rather than the 60 to 70 percent in the above formula. "They also have to watch their palpitations and things like that, and should first discuss the cardiotoxicity and precautions with their doctors." She also points out that patients shouldn't do anything too vigorous if their platelet counts dip below 30,000 because they could bleed into their joints, and she warns against taking dangerous risks involving balance which may be off due to the drugs.

Exercising three or four times a week is the goal in most programs, but if you can't attain this all the time, remember that something is better than nothing. Chemotherapy patients often have good days and bad days. When you are having a bad day, says Maryl Winningham, "do something moderate rather than nothing at all. Give your body a break."

MASSAGE

A good massage is therapeutic for both the mind and the body. It is relaxing, it stimulates the circulation, it releases the joints, and it soothes away tension accumulated in the muscles.

Massage is a particularly useful, though temporary, way of easing the discomfort of a particular physical problem, of physical exercise, or of everyday living. Though massage is not a cure, it can relieve aches and pains and thus reduce or eliminate the need for some medications.

Denver Presbyterians' Pam Felling says, "A lot of people in the cancer ward have a masseuse come in from outside. It is offered to them for relaxation, pain relief, improvement of circulation—all the normal things that massage is good for. They get the same benefits that anyone would—they're not that different."

One possible difference in the danger of massage spreading a cancer, a question that is brought up in the massage textbooks. About this possiblity, Lin Perkin says, "With really deep massage in the area of a tumor, you can actually physically break off tumor cells into the increased circulation. It used to be thought that the increased circulation itself was carrying off more tumor cells, but now doctors are using hyperthermia in conjunction with chemotherapy and rather than spread the cancer, the increased circulation enchances the effects of the drugs. So it's more the mechanical effects of massage that are dangerous. I don't think a light massage would do any harm; nor would a massage that avoids the area of the tumor or in cases where the tumor has been removed."

Concerned patients should still check with their oncologists to determine whether massage should be light or deep. Massage should not be painful, although in shiatsu the sensation has been described as "a good hurt." Communicate with the masseur or masseuse too—let the therapist know whether you can tolerate only light stroking or a rubdown or whether you want something with more "oomph."

Massage therapy is available from professionals whose skills and manner vary; some states require licensing to ensure a certain level of ability. Your doctor, nurse, or social worker may know of a practitioner or may also refer you to a physical therapist who can give you a medical massage. When a massage is given by a family member or friend—no matter how amateur or brief—it can be a reassuring form of physical and emotional communication that closes any gaps between caring and doing. As one patient said, "Massage is one of the nicest things one person can do for another."

Side Effects

CHAPTER 10

Bone Marrow/ Blood Effects

The cells of the blood, which are manufactured in the bone marrow, reproduce rapidly and frequently and so are quite vulnerable to chemotherapy drugs. Almost all the drugs used in cancer chemotherapy affect these cells. The drugs that depress, or lower the activity of, the bone marrow are called *myelosuppressive* drugs.

The bone marrow produces three types of cells; the red blood cells which carry oxygen to the tissues of the body; the platelets which help the blood clot and control bleeding; the white blood cells which help fight infections. Low blood counts therefore affect you in three main ways: low red blood counts (*anemia*) leave you tired, weak, and listless; low platelets (*thrombocytopenia*) mean your blood cannot clot properly; too few white cells (*leukopenia*) make you more vulnerable to infection. All three counts can and do drop simultaneously; this is called *pancytopenia*. Blood counts generally are at their lowest level seven to ten days after a treatment, and at this point you are at the greatest risk of developing complications. Low blood counts are expected in most chemotherapies, and your oncologist will periodically order blood tests, called complete blood counts (CBCs), to use as the main guide in determining whether there should be any changes in the dosage and/or scheduling of the drugs. Your body has an enormous capacity to churn

147

out new blood cells, but not a great enough one to completely forestall the side effects. As a result, most chemotherapy patients will have blood-related side effects in varying degrees. If the counts dip too low, the treatment will be cut down or held back until the counts return to safer limits. In cases of severe myelosuppression, patients are observed very closely, perhaps in the hospital, and transfusions of blood cells may be given. But there are many precautions and special steps that you can take both to minimize the side effects and to prevent complications from setting in.

TIREDNESS AND WEAKNESS
(Low Red Cell Count)

For many chemotherapy patients, an ever-present tiredness is the toughest side effect to contend with. Though it tends to come and go in cycles, with the worst days usually right after a treatment, the listless feeling may never really disappear completely. This is how one person describes it:

> "It was like they were shooting an A-bomb into me that blew me away every time. The two weeks I was off chemo I spent getting myself back on my feet again. But I never really had the chance to say, 'Gee I feel great'— by the time I got to feel human again it was time to go back. It would have been nice to feel what it was like to be normal again just for a minute."

I am normally full of energy, the instigator of escapades (or easily talked into them), but on chemo I did a lot of staying at home. This state of not being quite myself was probably the most demoralizing side effect I had to live with. You think "Who is this person?" The tiredness of chemo is not an ordinary tiredness and rather hard to describe. It's more oppressive than coming home from a rough day on the job or staying up all night. I'd hear other people complain, "I'm so tired," and think "If you only *knew*!"

Sometimes it felt like the day before a cold or the flu arrives: a vague, allover dragginess, like car running on the wrong fuel. Mornings were usually the worst; I'm not a morning person to begin with, but some days it was so hard to get started that my husband had to help drag me out of bed, even though I knew that I would probably feel better once I was up and about. Other times it seemed I spent whole days sluggishly moving, dreamlike, through air as thick as water, my limbs made of lead, the very cells of my body made of stone. Chemo sometimes sapped me of the energy to walk, to think, to hold a pencil or a conversation, so overpowering was the heaviness in my mind, my bones, my guts, and my soul. The day after a treatment I'd find myself face down on a friend's couch, or under the covers of my bed, and unable to do anything but complain.

When the weakness was bad, it was very bad; when it wasn't, it was bearable. I did manage to continue to work the whole time I was on chemo—I completed one book in progress, wrote another, and delivered the finished manuscript the same week I wrapped up my chemo. I continued a modified exercise regimen. And I did socialize and have fun—went to dinner, parties, dancing, movies and so on—but I coordinated these outings with my "up" periods, those times when I felt nearly normal, and then I was almost hyperenergetic, as if to make up for lost time.

Though individual, my experience was not unique. "I think the biggest thing that people complain about is being tired," says Donna Park, assistant director of Nursing, Ambulatory Care, at New York's Memorial Sloan-Kettering. She points out that in spite of the expected tiredness, people, especially the women on adjuvant breast chemotherapy, are encouraged to "carry out their current life-styles" while on chemotherapy. However, she adds, "As health professionals we had at first underestimated the impact of this treatment on patients' daily lives."

This feeling of "general malaise," as the textbooks call it, though hardly life threatening, is the side effect that is nevertheless most likely to turn a cancer patient's life upside down. A constant lack of energy is what keeps people from living more normal lives, from doing all the things that they want or need to do, from feeling like themselves.

Much of the anxiety about the tiredness is related to the issue of working. Showing up at the job every day like everybody else can be a real problem about which not much can be done specifically, unless you have an understanding employer, terrific insurance, an undemanding job, or can make your own hours.

Still, many people who need to continue to work do manage

to muster up enough strength to get there and get through the work day. So much of our identities and sense of accomplishment are tied up with what we do, and it is this, combined with the necessity of earning a living, that drives us to get up and out in spite of the gargantuan effort it sometimes takes. One patient recounts:

"I got very tired when my blood count went too low. The lack of energy . . . I'm back to my normal habits now, but it took a while. I'm not one to sleep beyond seven or eight, even on my day off; on chemo I'd stay in bed until ten. Usually I'm at work by seven-thirty every morning; on chemo I got calls at eight-fifteen asking, 'Are you coming to work today?' Twice that happened. Then I got myself two alarm clocks. They were good about it at work, but I was mortified. By three in the afternoon, I sat there not moving, thinking 'I want to go home.' My staff knew it and understood. Usually, I work like a dog."

Sister Rosemary Moynihan, a social worker supervisor at Memorial Sloan-Kettering, tells of an amazing lady with a brain tumor who would call the same taxi every morning to drive her to work. She was very weak and would get dizzy and she couldn't do too much bookkeeping anymore, but the people at her work were her support system. She would mobilize to go to work every single day until two weeks before she died.

Sister Rosemary Moynihan believes the ability to continue to work during chemotherapy can be a major emotional and social support in helping a person to cope. She feels it has to do with the opportunity to reach out beyond oneself, to have a broader identity, to feel able to master things. She adds:

"Of course for a patient who works as an interior designer and has to look good and be on top and be present at odd hours—that's tough turf. People who have jobs where there is physical stress—people who operate heavy machinery or who are in sales and always have to be 'up' and 'on'—and people in high-powered executive positions find working difficult. But if you have a job with flexibility, where your appearance doesn't have primary importance and you can have one day up and one day down, you do better."

Overwhelming tiredness affects people's social and home lives too. Friends and family may not realize how tired and awful you feel; without any outward signs or symptoms, this is a side effect that others easily forget or are skeptical about. They may mistake your lack of enthusiasm for laziness, or as a sign of depression, or unsociability. It is important for you to make the effort to keep contact with the people you care about and to continue to do the things you like and need to do. It should be explained to people that you still want to spend time with them, but maybe not as often, or for as long, or in doing the same things you used to. You may need to learn how to get around the fatigue by, for instance, making some changes, setting priorities, and taking naps. Here is how several patients felt about this:

"I was exceptionally tired while I was on chemo; I had been the type of person who took on two jobs and worked sixteen hours. When I was on chemo, I worked one job and would come home and have to take a nap if I was going to be able to cope with the evening's activities."

"I was more tired than usual. In the afternoons I almost always had to lie down and take a nap. Then I was able to get right back into everything. Right back into my painting, right back into the choir, right back into other activities I enjoyed before."

"I used to come home from work and clean—I don't do it anymore, I have help once a week. Now I clean in the morning when I have most of my strength, because when I come home in the afternoon I can't do it. I wake up an hour earlier just to get the house straightened out so at least when I come home, everything is neat and clean."

At first, I'd lie around the apartment in the evenings being so *bored* and miserable. I was used to an active life, but I had to save what energy I had for work during the day. How much can you read? How much TV can you watch? About three months in the chemo I decided this would be the perfect time to do something I'd always wanted to do: learn a musical instrument. It was just active enough, kept my mind busy, and really gave me a sense of accomplishment.

Fatigue is largely due to anemia, or a lack of oxygen-bearing red blood cells. The cells of your body literally become starved for oxygen and function suboptimally. Feeling dizzy, chilly, short of breath, and having a tendency to become upset more easily than usual are also indications of anemia.

Fatigue may also be caused or contributed to by the accumulation of waste products that are produced when large numbers of cells are killed by chemotherapy, by a poor diet, by a lack of sleep, and by the emotional stress of coping with cancer and chemotherapy. Factors such as boredom, pain, and a lack of exercise may exaggerate the feeling of listlessness. Advanced cancer itself can make you tired.

Marguerite Donoghue and her co-authors list these additional signs of fatigue in *Nutrional Aspects of Cancer Care*: irritability, tearfulness, decreased ability to make decisions, withdrawal, apathy, feelings of hopelessness and helplessness, impaired concentration and memory, psychomotor retardation or agitation, increasing insomnia, lack of appetite, thoughts of suicide. These are all serious impediments to living a full, enjoyable life.

COPING WITH FATIGUE

"There's no simple, easy solution to tiredness," says Donna Park. But there are many ways to help you lessen, prevent, and learn to live with it.

· Check your diet to make sure it is nourishing. You may need to increase your intake of protein and carbohydrates or to take nutritional supplements: Some doctors may recommend iron or vitamin supplements to help build up your red cell count.

· Make sure to drink plenty of fluids to prevent accumulation of cellular waste products, the by-products of chemo.

· Plan your days' activities and take advantage of ways to save your energy—either by figuring out easier means by which to do them yourself or by getting someone else to do them. Sometimes your family or friends will be glad to pitch in, sometimes not. Outside household helpers can make all the difference during those times you just can't do what's needed—and some social agencies will help pay for this service. Many patients dislike asking for help from anyone, friend or stranger, but sometimes having help is the only way to get things done:

"I didn't do much housework at all. If you could have seen my place, you would have said, 'Oh I see how she managed.' I didn't do the dishes until hours after dinner was over. My mother was a great deal of help, but the rest of my family did not cooperate in this area. Someone came in to help once in a while."

"I was so debilitated that my husband and daughter were assuming some household responsibilities, and we had someone come in during the weeks I was on chemo. You spend two or three days a week throwing up and it's gonna knock you out."

"The worst part is the lack of energy. Needing the care of other people. It is embarrassing. It makes me feel old. People do things for old people. If you're independent as I am, you're used to doing things for yourself—and it's hard. I feel guilty when others do the work for me."

· Set reasonable goals and priorities; conserve energy for those tasks you must or prefer to do yourself. Keep safety in mind—accidents tend to happen to those who are tired or weak. Perform as many day-to-day activities as you can. The activity is beneficial and helps you maintain a sense of normality, independence, and self-esteem. "Make a choice about what activities you're going to do," advises Donna Park. Speaking of patients with advanced diseases, she says, "One of my pet things is that when people came into the clinic they're a little bit short of breath and tired. So I say, 'Please use a wheel chair.' For them it's like giving in. And I'll say to them, 'Don't waste your energy here. Save it. Wait till you get home.'"

· Rest when you are tired, especially before and after a chemo-therapy treatment. Or avoid trying to do too much after a chemotherapy treatment—pace yourself. No one should expect you to be Superman or Wonder Woman. Many patients find that short naps in the afternoon work wonders.

· Get more sleep—deep, restful, uninterrupted sleep if possi-ble. You may require more hours of sleep than you used to, so don't go by the old days. Go to bed earlier and/or get up later, whichever is more convenient. To help yourself sleep, you may want to take a tranquilizer or a sedative. But before trying this, many patients find these tips helpful: Maintain a regular bedtime schedule and ritual; keep your environment quiet and calm, without distractions; use relaxation techniques; and try to find the cause of any sleep-disturbing anxieties and fears and alleviate them. Dr. William Grace of New York City's St. Vincent's Hospital, says:

> "If the patient is on glucocorticoids [such as prednisone], which will keep some people on a little bit of a high, we recommend that they take this medication in the morning. This way, they don't get the same "high" and insomnia they usually get if they take it at night. Some patients use Dexatrim to counteract some of the fatigue. There are even some patients for whom we prescribe Dexedrine for chemotherapy-related fatigue. If you give it carefully, in small doses, it is safe, and many patients are able to continue working and lead more normal lives."

· Begin a mild exercise program which may be intensified eventually. Walk, do errands, and do light work around the house. In the right amounts exercise energizes you—it doesn't tire you out.

· Begin or resume a favorite hobby or activity to alleviate boredom. It's best to have some degree of productive work or employment while you are on chemotherapy because it makes life more fun and keeps you from dwelling on cancer, chemotherapy, and how crummy you feel.

POOR BLOOD CLOTTING
(Low Platelet Count)

When your platelet count drops, the ability of your blood to clot is reduced. Because there are other coagulation factors in the blood, most of them produced by the liver and rarely affected by chemotherapy, the blood will still be able to clot eventually, only the process will take longer than usual.

Your oncologist will know from your blood test whether your platelet count is low. In between blood tests, you should watch out for signs yourself: red dots in the skin (*petechiae*), an abundance of black-and-blue marks, unusual bleeding from the nose or gums, or blood in the urine or bowel movements. These symptoms should be brought to the immediate attention of your physician.

When your platelet count is low, you should take precautions to protect yourself from any physical trauma that could cause bleeding. Take it easy and avoid dangerous situations such as contact sports, heavy physical labor, or any violent jarring activity that could cause you to bleed in your joints. Wear protective gear during gardening and cooking and other potentially hazardous activities. Be careful with knives, scissors, and razors. Even blowing your nose forcefully can damage delicate blood vessels and cause bleeding. Doctors advise you not to take aspirin because it further diminishes the blood's ability to clot, so use an aspirin substitute such as Tylenol or Datril. Use a soft-bristled toothbrush and avoid flossing if you find your gums bleed easily. Sometimes switching from a wet razor to an electric razor is advised.

If you should injure yourself in spite of taking precautions, help the clotting process along by putting a clean cloth or paper towel over the wound and applying pressure for five or ten minutes. Elevate the affected part if possible, and use ice or cold water to constrict the blood vessels. Since a low platelet count is often accompanied by a low white cell count, take careful antiseptic measures to help prevent infection. If the bleeding hasn't stopped after twenty minutes, consult your doctor.

INFECTION (Low White Cell Count)

Colds and flu are the most common infections that chemotherapy patients have to worry about. These are definitely unwanted additional problems, but they rarely progress beyond the nuisance stage:

> "I did get a lot more colds than I usually got. My oncologist gave me a flu shot and ordered me to stay home from work because he was afraid I might get it during the 'High Holy Days' of the flu. He still insists I get a flu shot every year, even though my white blood count has never dropped as low as before and is fine now."

"If anybody came in his house and *sneezed*, I picked the infection up. One weekend I caught a cold from my daughter. The next Monday I was due for a treatment which my doctor wouldn't let me out of. So that day, there I was lying in bed with the shivers, I couldn't breathe, my chest and nose were killing me, and I was throwing up. I was a sight."

But the danger of infection can go beyond these minor respiratory diseases. Infections are the major causes of illness and death in cancer patients. Almost any organ or part of the body can become infected, including most often the mouth, skin, lungs, urinary tract, rectum, and reproductive organs. These infections may be bacterial, viral, fungal, or protozoal in nature; they may be common ones, but a higher than normal proportion are exotic types.

Most are minor and can be treated successfully with antibiotics or other medication. Severe infections require more aggressive therapy which includes white blood cell transfusions. These transfusions may also be given as a precaution, before infection sets in, when the white blood count dips too dangerously low. Infections of the exotic type and infections that are particularly acute can occur in the people with the leukemias, because in these kinds of cancer the chemotherapy is intended to and does greatly reduce the number of white blood cells. Dr. William Grace says:

"People on chemotherapy are going to run a risk of infection. Patients must know the signs of infection, that if they get an infection they can die, and that they should inform the doctor right away if they suspect they might have an infection. Some patients 'don't want to bother the doctor.' They have to learn to bother us. If they have a fever on Monday but don't call the doctor until Wednesday, it may be fatal or it may take them weeks in the hospital to recover from the infection. We now have very good oral antibiotics and can often keep patients out of the hospital if mild infections are detected early."

SYMPTOMS OF INFECTION

There are certain general signs of infection that you should watch out for and immediately report to the oncologist or nurse.

- Temperature of 100° F or higher
- Chills, shivering
- Loose bowels for longer than two days
- Burning sensation during urination
- Coughing, sore throat, chest pain, or shortness of breath
- Unusual discharge or blood from the urinary tract, lungs, rectum, vagina, and so on

In addition, patients should pay attention to the visible, accessible parts of the body that are most prone to infection. Since the immune system is impaired, the usual, normal signs of infection—redness, pus, and swelling—are not present or may not be apparent because these are actually signs of the body trying to fight the infection. In cases of severe immunosuppression, or of suspected infection, the oncologist may request tests of the urine, sputum, feces, and the nose, ear, and throat secretions.

INFECTION PREVENTIVE MEASURES

- Maintain a good nutritional status—eat a higher calorie, high protein diet. Vitamin/mineral supplements may be advised, especially vitamin C which many oncologists are prescribing for their patients. Drink two to three quarts of fluid every day.

- Check with your doctor about what foods to eat during your therapy. For example, Dr. Philip Pizzo, chief of Pediatric Oncology at the National Cancer Institute, suggests that chemo patients check with their doctors about the advisability of eliminating fresh raw fruits and vegetables at certain points in their therapy—such as when the white cell count is particularly low, or during a course of antibiotics. These foods may be potential sources for harmful organisms which can migrate from the gastrointestinal tract to other parts of the body and cause serious infection. "Normally these bacteria go in one end and pass uneventfully out the other," he explains, "but in chemo patients this may not be so."

- Observe good rules of hygiene. Bathe or shower daily if possible; wash hands before meals and sexual activity, and before and after visits to the bathroom. Keep your hands away from your face, your fingers out of your mouth, nose, and eyes.

- Avoid crowds and particularly people or children with infectious diseases. Avoid exposure to people with herpes, chicken pox, and measles—even if you had these infections in the past.

- Avoid exposure to bird and animal excreta—let someone else clean up the mess.

- Stop smoking and avoid smoky rooms. Take deep breaths of clean air occasionally.

- Get some exercise daily (aerobic exercise may help stabilize your immune system) but don't become overly fatigued. Get enough sound sleep and/or rest as needed.

- Avoid bar soaps—they are excellent mediums for growth of organisms. Use liquid dispenser and/or moisturing soap.

- Keep your skin in good condition—dry thoroughly after washing and moisturize it if it's dry.

- Guard against burns, scrapes, punctures, and cuts; take proper care of them if they do occur. Wear protective gear when gardening, washing, and cooking. Be cautious while shaving—switching to electric shavers is recommended.

- Maintain cleanliness and proper lubrication during sexual activity. Avoid excessive friction; prevent rectal contamination.

Sometimes antibiotics are used prophylactically. Dr. Grace remarks:

"We identify the people who seem to be at high-risk for infection—either due to their disease or their therapy—and treat them during their low white blood counts with preventive antibiotics that are known to reduce the risk of infections. These are most commonly used in patients with leukemia, but there's no reason not to use them in high-risk patients with other cancers."

SPECIAL PRECAUTIONS FOR WOMEN

The vaginal infections that plague women can be especially bothersome during chemotherapy, when lowered resistance joins forces with an altered hormonal/vaginal chemistry and less than optimum eating habits. There are several ways you can help protect yourself from these infections.

· When antibiotics are taken for a bacterial infection anywhere in the body, good bacteria are killed along with the bad ones, and in their absence fungus can take hold and flourish. To prevent this, many doctors recommend taking yogurt orally or as a douche to restore healthy bacteria in the body. Liquid acidophilus, available in health food stores, is a more concentrated source of friendly bacteria and may be used instead of yogurt. Using an antifungal vaginal medication may also be advised while you are taking antibiotics.

· Chemicals irritate and inflame delicate tissues and they upset the chemical balance of the vagina. Avoid feminine hygiene sprays, commercial douches, and deodorized tampons and napkins.

· Do not use an IUD for birth control; ask your doctor about safer alternatives. Change tampons frequently during menstruation and substitute napkins as often as possible, especially overnight.

· Watching your diet may help you cut down on vaginal infections. Though this has not yet been scientifically proven, many nutritionally oriented health professionals recommend cutting down on sugars and other refined carbohydrates because an overabundance of sugars in the vaginal tract can trigger yeast infections. Fungus-related foods that contain mold or yeast (cheese, beer, wine, vinegar, and breads) should be avoided.

· Your clothes can contribute to a higher incidence of infections. Wear cotton panties or ones with a cotton crotch. Avoid tight pants and prolonged wearing of synthetic exercise clothes or wet bathing suits.

· Maintain scrupulous cleanliness in the genital area. Make sure to wipe from front to back after bowel movements to avoid fecal matter entering the vagina.

CHAPTER 11

Gastrointestinal Effects

The gastrointestinal (GI) system, which includes the mouth and teeth, throat, esophagus, stomach, intestines, and rectum, is lined with cells that reproduce rapidly. These are therefore prime targets for anticancer drugs. Chemotherapy drugs also affect other organs that in turn influence the activity of the organs of the gastrointestinal tract. In addition, certain psychological factors such as fear, anxiety, and depression can affect both the digestive process itself and the way you feel about food, as can disruptions in your life-style and daily routine:

"I still cook for the family, that doesn't bother me. But a lot of times I'd rather not eat at all, just go to bed instead."

"I'd go to the cafeteria for lunch, get a bowl of soup, and think maybe I could eat. Once one of my co-workers came by and said in a friendly way, 'Hello dear.' I don't remember what was on his tray, but whatever it was, the smell just made me jump up and run out because I thought I was going to vomit. He didn't know I was on chemo and when I later explained, he said, 'That's alright. It's just that nobody ever turned green in front of me.'"

"I could only eat light breakfasts the days of my treatments. I was so worked up psychologically—knowing
what I was going to go through a few hours later—that
if I looked at food those mornings it would make me
sick."

A change in eating habits and preferences can affect your
life in many ways. I think what bothered me most about the
change in eating habits was first, that I love food, and second,
that eating is such a social event. I had to choose restaurants
very carefully, and eat differently from usual. Thanksgiving
was especially trying, since my mother makes a huge, scrump-
tious dinner. All that food, that rich food. Friends and relatives
eventually understood that I couldn't eat that much, and that
plain food was the best for me. But it still made me feel guilty
and like the odd man out. It was like being on a reducing diet
and feeling sick at the same time—it wasn't really by choice
that I couldn't join in the gastronomic fun. One of life's greatest
pleasures was taken away from me.

Clearly, many of chemotherapy's side effects occur in the
gastrointestinal system. The most common are nausea, vomiting, loss of appetite, and weight loss. In addition, chemotherapy can also cause bloating, constipation, dehydration, dental
problems, diarrhea, dry mouth, esophagitis (a sore, irritated
throat), heartburn, indigestion, milk intolerance, pain, stomatitis (a sore, irritated mouth), swallowing difficulty, taste
blindness, and weight gain. In addition, drugs can change the
way in which nutrients are absorbed, metabolized, utilized, and
excreted.

The side effects can alter both the amounts and types of
food eaten as well as the way the body handles the nutrients
that are being ingested. Patients on chemotherapy can easily
become malnourished to one degree or another. However, a
well-nourished patient has been shown to tolerate treatment
better, respond to treatment more favorably, recover from individual treatments more rapidly, maintain desirable weight,
feel better, and remain more active. (See chapter 8). It is ironic
that at the very time a patient needs to be highly nourished he
or she is undernourished because of the therapy. Sometimes
the toxicity to the gastrointestinal system is so severe that the
chemotherapy plan will be modified, but since the toxicity is
usually not at a life threatening level, oncologists generally are

reluctant to do this. Luckily, there is some headway being made in understanding, alleviating, and preventing many of these side effects through watching what and how the patient eats. Many of the suggestions can be carried out by the patients themselves, their families, and their friends. (A dietician, nutritionist, or nutrition-oriented physician or nurse can give a nutritional evaluation and more individual advice.)

Living conditions and the presence or absence of friends and relatives can make a big difference in how easily you are able to overcome your side effects and maintain a healthful diet. If you are being treated as a hospital inpatient, you are assured on the one hand of having food of at least a minimum level of quality and quantity. On the other hand, you forfeit a certain amount of control over what and when you eat. Mealtimes can be quite lonely, sterile, affairs because most hospitals do not have communal dining areas. Meals are served in large portions, three times a day, but most chemotherapy patients do better with small, frequent meals. Hospital food is notoriously unappetizing and it may also be of a different type from what you are used to: Very few institutions take into consideration the ethnic background and cultural preferences of their patients. It is not surprising that malnutrition has been found in 30 to 40 percent of hospital patients, and that the percentages are even higher in cancer patients. Friends and relatives can be especially supportive in this area by bringing in some of your favorite foods (after checking with hospital authorities) and by scheduling their visits around mealtimes so you have company while you eat.

If you are being treated as an outpatient or by a physician in private practice, you may be living at home or staying at a hotel, motel, rented apartment, or with friends or relatives. In these cases you should be able to have a certain amount of control over your food and its preparation—possibly over whole meals or parts of them, and/or between-meal snacks. It is important to buy and prepare wholesome fresh foods instead of settling for poorly prepared fare such as "fast foods." Friends and family can help out here too, whether or not they normally are responsible for preparing the meals in your family.

The National Cancer Institute, among others, has published booklets that deal specifically with gastrointestinal problems that result from cancer and chemotherapy. Many contain additional tips to those suggested here, plus recipes for special diets such as bland diets, blenderized foods, high-protein diets, low-fat or low-fiber diets, liquid diets, and so on. (See "Sources" for listing.)

NAUSEA AND VOMITING

Most chemotherapy drugs cause some degree of nausea and vomiting after injection or administration. Some drugs, however, are notorious for their ability to cause these reactions in a high percentage of patients. According to an article by Drs. W. F. Maule and M. C. Perry, a high potential for nausea and vomiting exists in the intravenously administered drugs: cisplatin, cyclophosphamide, daunorubicin, doxorubicin, dacarbazine, mechlorethamine, and streptozocin; a moderate potential exists in the IV forms of cytarabine, carmustine, methyl-CCNU, etoposide, Methotrexate (high dose), and mitomycin, and in orally administered lomustine and procarbazine. The other commonly used drugs have low potential to induce vomiting. We don't know why some drugs in particular cause more vomiting than others—as a group they neither have any other attribute in common nor do they differ significantly from other chemotherapy drugs that do not cause vomiting.

The intensity, onset, and duration of nausea and vomiting that a patient experiences from a drug depend upon the individual patient, his or her nutritional status, the dose of the drug, the rate of administration, and the presence of other drugs. Psychological factors have also been implicated, especially in the case of anticipatory vomiting before the drug is actually given. Basically, patients may experience nausea and vomiting that begin within a few hours after a treatment but are short-lived; nausea and vomiting that last for twelve to twenty-four hours; or a constant, low-level nausea that persists throughout the course of treatment but does not lead to vomiting.

Usually the onset of nausea and vomiting is delayed a few hours—from three to four, possibly up to twelve after administration. In some drugs it is swifter—as soon as a few minutes after injection. Those who experience a constant, low-level nausea may find a heightening of this sensation soon after a treatment. Though reactions can vary somewhat from treatment to treatment, a patient's reaction (unless treated) to the same drug is usually fairly consistent. A violent vomiter will not suddenly begin to experience persistent non-productive nausea or vice versa. Two people describe their usual reactions:

> "About four or five hours after my treatment the puke attack would begin. It went like this: The first one usually wasn't so bad because I'd have something in my stomach to throw up. Then I would throw up every twenty minutes for the next hour. Gradually they would get closer and closer together—every fifteen minutes, every ten minutes, every five minutes—by which time it was the dry heaves, pure bile. Then it would gradually slow down to every ten minutes, fifteen, twenty. Then would come the final one—I'd always know it was the final one. I'd put one hand on my forehead, one on my stomach, and breathe a big sigh of relief. Then I'd go to bed and sleep."

> "I never threw up, I was just nauseous the five days that I was on the chemo. I'd work all day in the hospital without eating; I couldn't—I didn't want to vomit. Because once I started, I was afraid I wouldn't ever stop. The nausea was even worse when other patients got sick themselves. That was awful."

My own particular reaction was the constant, low-level nausea. Though it rarely went away and would heighten at certain periods during my therapy, it was never bad enough to make me throw up—but I seldom throw up anyway and am able to count on the fingers of one hand the number of times in my entire life I've been sick to my stomach.

Because nausea and vomiting are so unpleasant, they are often the side effects that patients most fear. Vomiting can also become one of the most serious from a medical point of view. Deleterious results of prolonged, regular chemotherapy-induced nausea and vomiting include intolerance of the treatment, a generalized weakness, serious weight loss, loss of substances vital to the body such as water and nutrients that lead to malnutrition, dehydration, and electrolyte imbalance which brings on irritability, lethargy, convulsions, and respiratory and heart problems. Though this is extremely rare, vomiting is sometimes so violent and prolonged that ribs and vertebrae have been fractured, and the delicate tissue in the digestive tract has been torn.

Nausea and vomiting, therefore, jeopardize the successful

treatment of cancer and reduce the quality of life. According to the aforementioned Drs. Maule and Perry, a recent survey of fifty-six oncology centers revealed that up to 10 percent of patients who potentially could have been helped by chemotherapy refused it because of actual or anticipated nausea and vomiting. Dr. Richard Gralla of Memorial Sloan-Kettering thinks that "of acute, drug-induced side effects, nausea and vomiting are the leading problems." (He points out, however, that psychological problems of other nonacute nonimmediate side effects may be bothering patients more.) He says:

> "Basically, I think the main thing is with the quality of life. If the quality of life is terrible, it makes it that much more difficult to come back for the chemo even though they know it's a good thing to take. Even if you make up your mind to go through with it, it still makes your life miserable."

THE CAUSES OF NAUSEA AND VOMITING

Though some drugs may irritate the digestive tract directly, this effect is thought to be only a possible contributing cause of the nausea and vomiting associated with cancer chemotherapy. Rather, the drugs are capable of somehow triggering the parts of the brain that control nausea and vomiting. It may be the drugs themselves that do this, or it may be the drugs causing a neurotransmitter in the brain to trigger the vomiting.

Nausea is a very common protective mechanism found in many species of animals. When you eat or drink something (the most likely ways for substances to enter the body), it gets into the bloodstream. There are certain receptors in the brain that are constantly sampling the blood. When harmful substances reach a certain level in the blood, it causes nausea. "When you take foreign substances in, there are very few ways you can get rid of them," explains Dr. Gralla. "One of them is by vomiting. Unfortunately, the body doesn't know that you didn't take chemotherapy by mouth but by injection."

Many other factors and conditions can produce nausea and vomiting in cancer patients, such as tumor pressure on the GI tract, metastases in the central nervous system, other drugs being taken, pain, and chemical abnormalities caused by the cancer or the treatment. It is important to determine whether there are any contributing underlying causes of nausea and vomiting because this can influence the measures used to alleviate them.

USING DRUGS TO CONTROL NAUSEA AND VOMITING

Drugs that cause vomiting are called emetics; the drugs used to control nausea and vomiting are called antiemetics ("emesis" being the medical term for vomit). The inability to deliver safe, effective consistently reliable antiemetics that are inexpensive and easy for outpatients to take has without a doubt been one of the more embarrassing and frustrating failings in the history of the cancer support system. Those most widely used so far have not only been disappointingly ineffective, but have rather undesirable side effects of their own—sedation being the most notable. It has been difficult to find drugs that suppress vomiting, partly because the portion of the brain that controls this function lies so close to the area that controls the heart and lungs. Anything that would interfere with vomiting could affect the functioning of these vital organs as well. In addition, as one researcher observed, "Nausea and vomiting have never been very popular research topics."

Dr. Richard Gralla, for whom antiemetics research *has* proved interesting, says that there has recently been an explosion of research in this area:

> "From 1960 to 1978 there were fewer than thirty studies done on the prevention of nausea and vomiting in cancer chemotherapy patients. There have been probably several hundred since that time. Now we have several helpful drugs. The other question is whether these newer drugs can be combined to lessen the side effects of the antiemetics and to increase their effectiveness. We are finding ways to do that. Of course we are concentrating on agents that cause the most nausea, like cisplatin. The results there have been pretty exciting. Several groups are working on the group of agents that are the second worst offenders, and then the group after that, and so on."

Dr. William Grace, an oncologist at St. Vincent's Hospital in New York, feels much of the problem lies in the way the available drugs are—and are not—used. Doctors are not well informed and don't sit down and take the time to "fine tune" their patients' therapies or to explain to them how to take their antinausea medication. "The common perception is that the disease makes you sick, the drugs make you sick, they're all going to be sick people," he says. "But that's not true. A lot of these things can really be done well. A lot of people are getting quite sick because there's not enough attention being paid to detail, to giving chemotherapy well."

CLASSES OF ANTIEMETICS

Until recently, a group of drugs called *phenothiazines* has been the mainstay of antiemetic therapy. The drugs in this category are Compazine (prochlorperazine), which may be taken orally, and Trilafon (perphenazine) and Torecan (thiethylperazine), both of which may be taken orally and administered intramuscularly or intravenously. These "old drugs" have not been very beneficial except in cases where the anticancer agents have a low or moderate potential for causing nausea and vomiting. They are being supplanted by other drugs that are probably going to turn out to be much more useful.

The butyrophenones, for example, are sometimes effective in patients who do not respond to the phenothiazines. This group of drugs includes Haldol (haloperidol), administered orally or intramuscularly, and Inapsine or Innovar (droperidol), administered intravenously.

A drug called Reglan (metoclopromide) belongs to a group of drugs called *dopamine antagonists*. Metoclopromide had for years been used in relatively low oral doses with little effect. But when it was used in high doses intravenously, in experiments by Dr. Gralla and others, it was shown to be highly effective against the side effects of cisplatinum, a drug that results in severe nausea and vomiting that had proved unresponsive to other antiemetics.

Corticosteroids, as a class of drugs, have been found to have antiemetic properties, although it is uncertain why. Corticosteroids such as dexamethasone (Decadron) and methylprednisolone in high doses have been found to give good results.

Sedative/hypnotics such as Valium and Dalmane have been used to reduce nausea in patients. Marijuana, a member of this class of drugs, also has been shown to be an effective antiemetic for some chemotherapy patients. In spite of its illegal status as a recreational drug, its therapeutic use for cancer patients has gained broader acceptance and gotten a lot of publicity. As a result, you may be able to get legal "joints" from your oncologist or capsules or suppositories containing THC, the active ingredient in marijuana. However, because of all the red tape involved, it is usually recommended that patients obtain this drug through nonmedical channels; in addition, as one oncologist confessed, "You can get much better grass on the street that you can from the state." My oncologist mentioned marijuana early on in the therapy and said he had no objections if I could get some and use it.

Though it does work for some people, marijuana is no panacea. Its side effects can vary considerably and they depend upon many factors including the strength of the drug and the patient's expectations and prior experiences. The side effects that might benefit cancer patients include the well-known "high" or sense of well-being, its relaxing and tranquillizing effects, an increase in appetite, and a lessening of pain. Marijuana, however, may also cause undesirable side effects such as paranoia, disorientation, an inability to concentrate, acceleration of the heartbeat, dry mouth, and red eyes. Be sure to check with your physician before taking marijuana if you are obtaining it through nonmedical channels; you may have a physical condition or be taking other drugs upon which marijuana might have an adverse effect.

These unpleasant side effects are particularly unacceptable in older patients, and many who have been given THC once have refused to take it again. Research is being conducted to develop synthetic THC that will have fewer side effects than the natural THC found in marijuana.

Patients find marijuana works best if they begin using it *before* a treatment and continue to use it regularly afterward until the time comes when they would usually stop vomiting. Three to five puffs begin to have effect in a few minutes and last for about two hours. When taken by mouth, in brownies or cookies, or as a capsule, the effect begins in forty-five minutes or two hours and lasts two to six hours. Marijuana is also available as rectal suppositories—when used this way, the effect begins in thirty minutes and lasts up to six hours.

More information may be found in *Using Marijuana in the Reduction of Nausea Associated with Chemotherapy* by Roger A. Rothman, assistant professor of Social Work at the University of Washington. In this book he describes the psychological and physiological effects of marijuana and how to acquire, prepare, and use it, including recipes for incorporating it in foods.

Antinausea drugs are far from perfect. Not all work as effectively as we'd like; some work better against some emetics than others. The drugs need to be taken hours before chemo is given (some recommend twenty-four hours) and then repeated at two-, three-, or four-hour intervals until the nausea is scheduled to subside. Oral antiemetics have the advantage of being self-administered by the patient, but they may be unreliable and only partially effective against many emetics, or for some drugs, unavailable in this form. Intramuscular or intravenous administration, the most effective mode for some high-dose antiemetics such as metoclopromide or corticosteroids, on the other hand, must be done by a trained professional, is time-consuming, and so is limited to hospital inpatients for the most part. In addition, there is the cost: Oral antiemetics may cost as little as $1.00 for twenty-four hours' worth of treatment, whereas twenty-four hours of metoclopromide given in the hospital costs nearly $200—in addition to the other costs of chemotherapy including the anticancer drugs themselves. None of the antiemetics are without side effects, with sedation being the most prevalent. Marijuana, although it falls somewhere in the medium-price bracket as an antiemetic, in many instances is purchased illegally and so poses its own additional unique disadvantages.

My oncologist gave me a prescription for Compazine when I started the chemo. But my reaction was a slight constant nausea, which heightened in waves without any warning. So I felt I never really needed the Compazine too badly—besides, I would have had to take it every day. I ended up never using it and throwing the pills away. I thought I was putting enough chemicals in my body as it was and decided to grin and bear it. I was one of the more fortunate ones in that I didn't have the severe reaction that necessitates the use of imperfect antiemetics that these patients experienced:

"I spent the year pretty much stoned. I smoked marijuana every time I went for a treatment; I also took Compazine at the same time. I don't know whether there was any effect or not, but I was afraid to try a treatment without that stuff. I had such a terrible time with it, what would I do if it were even worse without it? I didn't want to know."

"You wouldn't believe the drugs they gave me for the nausea. They tried everything on the market. First they tried Compazine. They tried it in different dosages, but that didn't work. They tried it in suppositories, but that didn't work either. Then they tried another drug. That didn't work. Finally they tried a new drug that came in a patch you put behind your ear; I'd start putting that on the night before they gave me the treatment. That didn't work either. They suggested I try marijuana. At first I didn't mind the idea of getting high for medical purposes. But then I thought, 'I've already had one kind of cancer. Now I'm going to start smoking something that might give me lung cancer just so I won't feel the side effects of cancer therapy? What am I, crazy?'"

"One of the amusingly frustrating aspects of my treatment had to do with marijuana. I felt I was cheated—I had heard about using grass to control nausea, and never having smoked controlled substances before, I was looking forward to this opportunity to try it. But they just gave me something through the IV along with the chemo that knocked me out."

The problems with antiemetics are far from completely solved, but there are ways of getting around them, and ways to enhance the drugs' effectiveness.

· *Timing*: Dr. Grace says, "You always start antinausea medication before you give the chemo. You've got to put the drug on the emesis center to change the emesis threshold. Once people start to be sick, forget it. It's very hard to stop it. The physician must use antiemetics prophylactically—he must have the pills around, or write the prescription, and explain to the patients how to take it. This is a very labor-intensive field and doctors must take the time to be compassionate." Dr. Ronald Bash also recommends that his patients begin taking an antiemetic several hours before a treatment. He favors prescribing them in suppository form because many patients tolerate them better than oral medication. In addition, anti-

emetics should be continued for a day or a day and a half
after the treatment, because nausea can persist this long.

Sedation, a common side effect of antiemetic drugs, can
limit your mental and physical activities. This disadvantage,
too, may be sidestepped by judicious use of timing and may
even become an advantage. Patients find it often helps if they
can sleep through the hours in which the worst nausea and
vomiting are likely to occur. The sedative effects of the antiemetics can help them to do this. In fact, tranquilizers, sed-
atives, and antihistamines have all been prescribed for their
antiemetic effects.

Those who are receiving chemotherapy as inpatients are
often given an intravenous antiemetic right through the same
IV that the chemo goes through. They then spend a whole
day and/or night sleeping. Outpatient treatments and antiemetics can also be scheduled so the patients sleep through
the worst of it. If you are home, try to have someone check
on you periodically because it is possible to vomit in your
sleep, inhale it, and suffocate. Elevating the head of the bed
either with pillows or a prop under the mattress will help
prevent this from occurring.

In addition, oral chemotherapy can all be taken at once,
in the evening, instead of throughout the day. If it is taken
along with an antiemetic and a sedative, patients sleep through
any nausea. Though there is a theoretical possibility that a
higher concentration of the drug in the urinary tract could
increase the risk of toxicity (cystitis), Dr. Grace doesn't see
this effect in his practice. "If patients drink a lot of water at
night, they wake up to urinate. The difference is infinitesimal;
patients just don't have urinary problems."

· *Type and Dosage*: You may need to experiment with drugs
and their amounts in order to hit upon the right antiemetic
therapy for you. It is odd that the most commonly used agent
for antiemesis in chemotherapy is Compazine, which, says
Dr. Grace, "is basically a mediocre antiemetic." When one
antiemetic doesn't work, you should switch to one of another
class, or increase the dosage, or combine drugs of different
classes. Just as combinations of cancer chemotherapy drugs
are usually more effective against cancer, combinations of
antiemetics work better than single agents. This approach can
also be helpful if an effective antiemetic begins to lose its
power. If patients get "breakthrough nausea"—a little more

nausea with each cycle because of the accumulative toxicity—
"the patient," says Dr. Grace, "might have to escalate the war.
You increase the dose or add another antiemetic."

"Because it is such a powerful emetic, cisplatinum is the
gold standard by which all antiemetics are judged," puns Dr.
Ronald Bash. This is why high-dose IV metoclopromide was
such a breakthrough. But it is expensive in IV form and it
must be administered in the hospital. Metoclopromide, however, can be taken in pill form, in high doses for highly toxic
drugs, and in lower doses that are effective for less toxic
drugs. "You can get the same high dosage as that in IV form,"
says Dr. Grace, "but it's a handful of pills that must be taken
every three hours. There are some people who can be given
chemotherapy and munch on handfuls of pills, but for others
the concept of swallowing pills—they can't do that. I'm not
recommending that taking ten to fifteen tablets is a great way
to get your dosage of antiemetic. But it has been done in at
least one study and has been found acceptable for a large
group of people who otherwise would have to be in a hospital."

At this moment in the history of chemotherapy, there is no
single, reliable antiemetic without side effects. In addition,
patients and their oncologists must therefore be willing to do
a bit of juggling and experimentation. Too, patients must decide
which side effects are most acceptable: those from the anticancer drugs or those from the antiemetics. Where effective
antiemetics do exist, most patients with severe reactions would
rather spend their time sedated instead of vomiting. Where
reactions are not so severe, the choice is not so easy. In those
cases where reactions are severe and the oncologists—for
whatever reason—have not found effective antiemetics, patients learn to sit tight and ride out the vomiting that occurs
after a treatment.

PSYCHOLOGY AND VOMITING

Nausea and vomiting can have a strong psychological component. The atmosphere and spirit in which chemotherapy is
given perhaps can play a role in how nauseated a patient gets,
as can the patient's expectations. Dr. William Grace feels
strongly:

"You can't have cancer patients come in and expect to get sick. From day one we tell them that with the proper antiemetics the probabilities are very remote. Also, people who get chemotherapy should get it in a private room which is warm and well-ventilated so that anybody who is sick in another room is neither heard nor seen by the patient. In some cancer centers, you sit in a room and everybody watches everybody else getting sick. You get a visual reinforcement that the stuff going in your arm is going to make you sick; there is also auditory and olfactory reinforcement. People like to talk to each other before and after, but getting chemo itself is, I think, a very private thing. I don't think they like to get chemo together, especially if something bad is happening."

In addition, chemotherapy patients can develop conditioned aversions to specific foods. This situation is illustrated by patients who learn to refuse certain foods because they associate them with the treatment and vomiting. There is a well-known study carried out in Seattle in which one group of children were given a particular flavor of ice cream just before a chemotherapy treatment. Another group was given the same flavor, but no treatment. A third group got chemotherapy, but no ice cream. The group that received the chemotherapy after the ice cream were the children who most often refused the ice cream when it was given again. This situation is very much like the conditioned response that Pavlov elicited from his dogs that learned to salivate at the sound of a bell because they associated it with being fed. One patient had a similar learning experience while on chemotherapy. "I couldn't keep anything down for a few days following the treatment, and my husband kept trying to give me foods like plain yogurt and soup. It took until months after I was off chemo to again start eating these things he gave me." Refusal of food becomes a conditioned response not related directly to the presence or absence of nausea; as a result, patients avoid certain foods or all foods throughout the therapy, not just during the time after therapy.

Another example of conditioning as a result of chemotherapy is called anticipatory nausea and vomiting. This occurs in about 25 percent of those taking chemotherapy, and is characterized by the patient feeling the side effect before the drugs could possibly have taken effect, often before they are even

administered. Some patients wake up nauseous on the day of
treatment, or they begin to feel symptoms on the way to the
doctor, or just as the needle is being inserted, or nonemetic
agents are being administered. Sometimes just seeing the physician, whether on a treatment day or not, passing by the hospital, or being in the same neighborhood as the clinic can trigger
nausea and vomiting. A patient remembers, "If I even smelled
rubbing alcohol, I would start retching from the association."
For this type of reaction, relaxation therapies are being used,
with encouraging results. Matthew Loscalzo, a social worker
who treats patients for this and other problems related to cancer
and chemotherapy at Memorial Sloan-Kettering in New York,
says:

> "Anticipatory nausea and vomiting is a conditioned aver-
> sion. Usually by the third or fourth session, upon waking
> that day the patient may vomit, just at the thought of
> going in to the hospital. One thing I do with patients is
> to let them know that this is at first a physiological re-
> sponse to the drugs. The body becomes nauseated and
> the patient learns to associate the entire environment of
> the hospital with the side effect. People tend to learn
> very quickly when they are under stress, or are emo-
> tionally depleted, or when their anxiety level is high.
>
> "It is not simply a psychological process—there is
> nothing psychologically wrong with you. You simply
> have to relearn something. It's in part a physiological
> process like learning to play the piano. After a while,
> your fingers play the piano and you don't have to think
> about it. It's the same with this."

Relaxation techniques are also being used to reduce post-
chemotherapy nausea and vomiting that result after a chemotherapy treatment has been given, though with not quite such
dramatic results. Mr. Loscalzo continues:

> "With postvomiting and nausea there's a good reason for
> people to be ill. Their bodies have been subjected to
> chemotherapy. It's very different from the conditioned
> aversion experienced before a chemo treatment. It can,
> however, also be exaggerated. We can help these people
> with their anxiety, but only up to a point. They are still

going to feel ill—that is normal. But we can help them to reduce some of the distress that they're feeling because they can control their anxiety."

This patient underwent relaxation and hypnosis to relieve her anticipatory nausea and vomiting:

"I was getting sick even before I had the treatment. One of the nurses mentioned that a doctor was using hypnosis for chemo patients and it seemed to work well. In the beginning I had five sessions a week with the hypnotherapist. This was disturbing because he was in the same building as my chemotherapist and the second time I went I got sick because of the association. My hypnotherapist assured me it would never happen again—and it didn't. I stopped having the anticipatory nausea and vomiting.

"He also tried to help me control the nausea after the chemo, but that he couldn't do completely. What did happen was that I was able to recover from the chemo faster. The nausea went away faster and I could eat sooner. He just suggested it to me while I was in the trance. He told me what was going to happen, what I should expect to eat. Within twenty-four hours I could handle light food."

M. L. Frohling, who uses these techniques at Denver Presbyterian Hospital, illustrates another example of how these techniques are used to control these side effects:

"There was one patient who had to be hospitalized for severe nausea and diarrhea. She was getting chemotherapy after surgery as a precaution. She didn't believe there was any cancer left in her body and she perceived the chemo as coming in and killing off only healthy cells. Through visual imagery I was able to help her realign her belief system to be more oriented toward regaining her health instead of thinking the chemo was destructive. Once her conflict was resolved, she had her third round of chemo without a bit of nausea."

NONDRUG MEASURES TO REDUCE NAUSEA AND VOMITING

Cancer professionals have devised many hints to help their patients reduce nausea and vomiting. You might want to try them if your nausea and vomiting are mild, or you don't want to take antiemetics, or you want to do something on your own to help reduce this side effect instead of or in addition to taking antiemetics.

· Methods of consuming foods and beverages that have worked under other nausea-inducing conditions such as illness, stress, or pregnancy may work in this case. For example, nausea in the morning may respond to remedies recommended for morning sickness—eating melba toast, dry toast, or crackers upon awakening and before getting up.

· It is important to avoid dehydration—drink plenty of water and other liquids, especially before and as soon as after a treatment as possible. Carbonated beverages such as ginger ale, 7-Up, or Coca-Cola can help curb nausea. Clear liquids such as fruit juices, clear soups, Popsicles, or gelatin desserts are usually tolerated.

· Bland, light foods—mashed potatoes, applesauce, sherbert, toast, yogurt, cottage cheese—stay down more easily.

· Avoid sweet, salty, greasy, and hot or spicy foods with strong odors.

· Eat foods cold or at room temperature to avoid releasing strong odors that can sometimes trigger nausea.

· Sometimes sour or tart foods—pickles, lemons, sour hard candy—or rinsing the mouth out with lemon juice and water help curb nausea.

· Always sip liquids and eat foods slowly. Avoid drinking during meals. Eat in a still, relaxed, quiet environment.

· Experiment with the amount and timing of your meals. For some patients, avoiding any food or drink for one or two hours before and after a treatment helps. Sometimes eating a large meal three to four hours before the treatment and eating lightly the rest of the day does the trick. If neither of these helps, try eating several small, light meals during the day.

· If the smell of food nauseates you, let others do the cooking and avoid the cooking area. Stick with foods that do not have strong odors.

· Ask to have the timing of your treatment changed—some patients report a decrease in nausea when the treatment is given early, others when it is given late in the day. The method of administration can sometimes make a difference: The slower drip (infusion) method can cut down on nausea.

· Oral chemotherapy that makes you nauseous can be taken along with food or milk and/or an antacid. This sometimes reduces nausea, but check with your physician to make sure there is no compatability between drugs.

· Distract yourself. Watch TV, go to the movies, or socialize to take your mind off nausea.

· Many patients report that exercise reduces nausea. As I mentioned in Chapter 9, this worked well for me and swimming worked best of all. However, activity after meals can increase your discomfort, and perhaps even trigger vomiting.

· Use relaxation techniques such as meditation, hypnosis, and visualization. Studies have shown that these therapies do help reduce nausea and vomiting in many patients (see Chapter 7) and are especially effective in anticipatory nausea and vomiting.

Many patients find that one or a combination of these methods helps them handle nausea and vomiting. Often they come up with tricks of their own—some of them bizarre—help them get through it:

"I tried to do something to occupy my mind, to talk myself out of feeling sick. I convinced myself that having a Coke and a doughnut before a treatment helped."

"I craved fruit juices. And I ate salty pretzels before a treatment—somehow they were not too unpleasant when I vomited and they stayed pretty much the same on the way up as on the way down."

"Chicken soup and toast were the only things I tried. But after a while, I didn't try anything. I'd wait until I came home from work, have a brandy, and get knocked out. I'd go to sleep immediately, and I guess that's why I thought it was the only thing I could tolerate."

"I smoked cigarettes while I was on chemo, though I don't anymore. They were my crutch. You'd think that they would have made me sicker, but every time I felt a wave of nausea, I'd light up and it went away. Maybe it was the deep breathing rather than the cigarette."

LOSS OF APPETITE, WEIGHT LOSS

Loss of appetite (anorexia) and the resulting weight loss are of primary concern during chemotherapy. Often it is complications due to malnutrition that lead to other illnesses, and possibly death especially in advanced cancer patients. Loss of five, ten, fifteen, and even more pounds are common, but they should be minimized or prevented if possible because patients do better and feel healthier and stronger physically and psychologically if their normal weight is maintained.

CAUSES OF APPETITE LOSS

Anorexia is one of the most difficult side effects to treat because it can have so many contributing causes. These include psychological and emotional factors, the disease itself, and its treatment. For example, depression, fear, and anxiety often cause people to lose their desire for food. These emotions can begin to take their toll early on: Patients who have been told that they might have cancer have been known to lose between five and ten pounds while waiting for a firm diagnosis! After diagnosis, emotions continue to affect the appetite and they don't stop during the ups and downs of treatment or if the disease recurs.

Side effects of chemotherapy such as mouth sores, diarrhea, constipation, malabsorption, lethargy, sleep disturbances, and alterations in the ability to taste and/or smell food also play their parts. So do changes in life-style such as isolation from other people or reduced physical activity. In addition, conditioned responses from nausea or pain due to treatment make the idea of food less appealing. Physical problems related to the location of a tumor (in cancers of the head, neck, esophagus, stomach, bowels) can affect ability to eat; surgery and radiation to these parts can cause difficulty in swallowing, dry mouth, pain, and problems with digestion and taste perception. The tumor itself, rapidly dying cells, or toxicity to certain organs such as the hypothalamus or liver can release chemical messages that interfere with the appetite.

HOW TO INCREASE FOOD INTAKE

Patients who are overweight at the start of their therapy often don't mind the expected weight loss. However, as explained in Chapter 7, it is important to keep well-nourished. In addition, weight loss can set off harmful chemical reactions in the body or may be interpreted as a sign that the disease is advancing. Health professionals do not like to see their patients lose weight at this time. Lisa Logan, clinical dietician at Denver Presbyterian Hospital, says, "The last thing I usually recommend for cancer patients is weight loss, no matter how much they weigh when I assess their conditions." Dr. Ronald Bash agrees: "Oncologists get scared when they see their patients losing weight. It's a bad sign in cancer. And you never know when a patient is going to need his or her weight."

There are many practices that can help increase or maintain your appetite and/or the amount of food you eat. Many are simple tips or tricks, some involve behavior modification, others rely on special products or foods to boost nutrition.

· You may need to change the meaning of food in your life. Instead of eating to satisfy your taste buds or your hunger, you may need to eat foods that seem tasteless and at times when you are not really hungry. A good deal of pleasure may be missing, but eating good, nourishing food is an integral part of your treatment.

· If possible, consult with a dietician and/or nutritionist who will explain what a balanced, nutritious diet contains and help you plan your daily menu. Take a few sample hospital menus home with you as examples when planning your own meals after you have been released. It may be advisable to add vitamin/mineral supplements to your diet to supply the nutrients that you are missing.

· Drink plenty of liquids and emphasize those with high nutritional content such as milk, milk shakes, and juices. Fruit nectars are high in calories and delicious.

· If appetite-depressing side effects such as pain, stress, tiredness, mouth sores, taste blindness, constipation, or diarrhea are present, try relieving them by using the methods recommended elsewhere in this book.

· Eat in a relaxing, pleasant atmosphere with soft music, good company, perhaps a glass of wine. It is helpful if friends and family encourage you, but they should understand that it is unwise to try to force to you eat at this time.

· What you eat is as important as how much. Although you should eat the foods you like, it may be wise to stay away from your favorite foods when you don't feel like eating. Patients often develop an aversion to foods eaten when ill, and then find them undesirable even when they feel well. It's better to stick with nonaromatic, cold foods about which you have neutral feelings, food such as juices, Popsicles, or gelatin desserts.

· Try to include as many highly nutritious foods as possible, especially in between treatments when your appetite is better. That's the time to indulge in your favorite foods, too. Patients often talk about making up for lost time by gorging in pizza or cheesecake after the nausea subsides. Donna Park thinks that "People are too strict with chemotherapy patients sometimes and insist that they eat something nutritious when they have no appetite for it. I'd rather they eat something that is maybe less nutritious but at least gets eaten. At least it has calories. So what if a patient eats ice cream three days a week?"

· Arrange to have your biggest meals whenever your appetite is at its best—this is usually in the morning, but it may be different for you.

· If you are too tired to shop and cook, ask friends and relatives to help out. During your "up" periods you can cook and freeze food portions that you can easily warm up and eat during your "down" times. Or rely on nutritious convenience foods such as creamed soups or "Lite" frozen dinners.

· Exercise before a meal can perk up a flagging appetite. Do simple range-of-motion exercises, walking, or anything you like and can manage for at least five or ten minutes one half hour before meals.

· Studies show that cancer patients can require up to hundreds of additional calories and twice as much protein as noncancer patients. However, many high-protein foods—meat particularly—are often repulsive to cancer patients; unfortunately many high-protein foods are also high in fat, which chemotherapy patients may have trouble digesting and are of questionable value healthwise. Many professionals, nevertheless, advise patients to try to add high-calorie, high-protein (and, often, coincidentally high-fat, high-sugar) foods and food supplements to their diets and usual recipes. These foods include butter, peanut butter, cheese, eggs, powdered milk or protein supplements (found in health food stores) added to milk, juice, shakes, or other prepared dishes, Instant Breakfast or Granola Bars, or eggnogs and milk shakes. Other sources of low-fat protein can be found by combining plant proteins with each other and with small amounts of fish, poultry, milk products, or meat. Vegetable protein, made from soybeans, can be added to ground meat dishes—this lightens them by reducing the fat content without sacrificing the protein.

SUPPLEMENTATION

In cases of severe weight loss, 5 percent or more of the total body weight, patients become "candidates" for nutritional supplements. There are commercially prepared high-protein, high-calorie food supplements available in liquid or pudding form. These "formulas" are available in drug stores and from home health care suppliers and can be used as substitutes for regular food or in addition to it. "These do tend to have an unpleasant aftertaste," admits Lisa Logan. "So I try to make them more palatable for the patient by adding ice cream, fruit, milk products, and eggs which mask the flavor and boost up the nutrients." Other possible additions include flavoring extracts, fruit juice, and carbonated beverages. These preparations are low-residue, however, and can lead to constipation.

Sometimes freezing liquid supplements and eating them like ice cream or blending them in a milk shake makes them more palatable.

In advanced cancer patients, when there is pronounced weight loss, weakness, and malnutrition, hyperalimentation may be used. The patient is fed with liquids containing vitamins, minerals, protein, fat, and other substances through tubes inserted into the gastrointestinal tract of the veins. Up to 4,000 calories can be taken in this way by patients who badly need them, and whose condition can improve remarkably because of this therapy.

TASTE BLINDNESS

Many chemotherapy patients experience a loss of taste or a change in the way foods taste, which occurs because the lining of the tongue and the chemical receptors that detect taste are altered. Patients often find that food tastes "different" or "bad." High-protein foods such as meat—beef and pork in particular—usually lose their appeal; it is thought that this low tolerance for meat stems from a lower threshold for bitterness because chemical imbalances in the body react to amino acids in the food. Patients have said, "I found myself gagging on certain foods, like steak," or "I didn't like meat at all—I'd cook for my family, but I wouldn't eat it myself."

Sweets can also seem less seductive than usual. Some researchers have found that patients have an elevated threshold for sweets up to a certain point. Once that point is reached, though, additional sweetness becomes intolerable. Many patients find in general that "nothing tastes right" and their appetites suffer. One patient remembers: "I didn't like anything sweet. My appetite wasn't normal; I usually just had one serving of what we were having, no seconds. I cooked still, that didn't bother me. Just the sweet stuff—cake, candy. I still baked for my husband, and it didn't bother me to see him have it; I just didn't want any for myself."

There are very few ways of getting around the alterations in taste that chemotherapy patients experience; the condition may be aggravated by a bad, metallic taste left in the mouth from certain drugs.

- Sometimes hypnotherapy and visualization help. (See Chapter 6.)

- Incorporate other, nonbitter high-protein foods if you find you have an aversion toward meat. Fish and poultry are usually still palatable, for instance; and dried beans, cheese and other milk products, eggs, and the complementary proteins found in beans, whole grains, and nuts can be made into many appetizing dishes.

- Protein supplements may be helpful. According to Earl Mindell, author of *Earl Mindell's Vitamin Bible*, the best ones are derived from soybeans. They supply complete protein and there is no danger of lactose intolerance. Protein supplements are available in liquid and powder form and usually supply twenty-eight grams of protein per two tablespoons—the same amount you get from a three-ounce steak.

- Add extra seasonings and spices to foods, if you tolerate them.

- Acid foods such as oranges and grapefruits tend to stimulate the taste buds, so include some with your meals.

- As when dealing with loss of appetite, attractively served, well-prepared food served in comfortable setting can be helpful in restoring (or ignoring) the way food tastes.

- A zinc deficiency can alter your ability to taste food; ask your physician about taking a zinc supplement.

WEIGHT GAIN/WATER RETENTION/BLOATING

The popular picture of the chemotherapy patient is someone who is sick, vomiting, not eating, and losing weight to the point of emaciation. Many patients do lose weight, but many others, particularly women on adjuvant chemotherapy for breast cancer, instead find themselves tipping scales in the opposite direction. This can be aggravated by or partially caused by an increase in appetite, water retention, and abdominal bloating. Even though I lost weight on chemo, I developed a little pot belly during the time I was on prednisone; this bloating disappeared when the drug was withdrawn. Many women, however, find it a real problem to lose weight they gained while on chemo that is not due to water retention. Donna Park says this weight gain can be "devastating."

> "The women are often gaining tremendous amounts of weight, so they have an altered body image not only because of the mastectomy, but because of the weight they gain. They put on fifteen, twenty, thirty pounds— it depends on how careful the patient is. We're not sure if it's only because of the prednisone. One of the theories we have is that patients are eating constantly to relieve their continuous nausea. Another theory is that they're feeling 'Well, I don't know what next year will bring, so I'm going to eat to make myself feel better.' Or it might be because they are engaged in less activity, so they burn fewer calories."

Prednisone and dexamethasone are corticosteroids given as part of several chemotherapy plans. Their side effects include an increase in appetite and salt and water retention. A diet low in salt and refined carbohydrates, and high in protein and potassium, is usually recommended to help keep weight gain and water retention to a minimum. Here are some tips to help keep the scales' numbers down.

· Do not add salt to foods that are being cooked and leave the salt-shaker off the table when you eat.

· Watch out for hidden salt in prepared and convenience foods. Avoid anchovies, bouillon, soups, canned fish, bacon, cold cuts, corned beef, frankfurters, sausage, potato chips, corn chips, pretzels, salted nuts, soy sauce, catsup, and hard cheeses. Look for salt-reduced versions of these products.

· Look for cookbooks with salt-reduced recipes and tips that help you lower your salt intake without sacrificing too much flavor. Use herbs, spices, and lemon juice to perk up recipes.

· If the problem persists or is severe, your doctor may prescribe a diuretic (a pill that rids the body of excess water). Some foods are natural diuretics: citrus juices, parsley, some herbs, and water itself. Exercise (swimming in particular) seems to act as a diuretic too.

· Eat foods high in potassium—bananas, apricots, cantaloupe, orange juice, potatoes—which cortisone depletes from the body, or take a potassium supplement. Using diuretics also depletes potassium.

One contributor to overweight are the binges that go on between treatments when the patient feels well, for example, "I'd lose weight for the five days I was on chemo, but the moment I stopped, I ate like a pig. I hate pizza normally, but I'd bring home a big pizza and just gorge myself. Ice cream, anything. Just to get rid of the memory of the nausea."

As Ms. Park mentioned, a constant nausea may drive you to constant nibbling in an effort to mask the unpleasantness; a bad taste in your mouth, a common side effect of many drugs, can do the same. Perhaps low calorie food items such as raw vegetables, fresh fruit, hard candy, fruit juices, ginger ale, or no calorie herbal teas will serve this function as well as more fattening foods.

According to Dr. Grace, some of his patients find that if they take their oral chemotherapy spaced out over the day instead of all at once, the slight nausea they get helps keep their appetite down. Some patients also take Dexatrim while on chemo—this not only curbs the appetite but counteracts some of the fatigue caused by the therapy. He suggests that if patients take a corticosteroid such as prednisone, they take it on alternate days instead of every day. "They don't get anywhere near the amount of bloating they usually get, even though they take the same total amount."

Eating to "make yourself feel better" because of anxiety about your prognosis or condition may be remedied by a talk with your oncologist or to the psychological/relaxation therapies described in Chapter 7. It's always preferable to prevent a weight gain than to have to lose it afterward as this patient discovered:

"One thing I was very down about was the way I ate— I put on thirty-five pounds while I was on chemo. I changed my eating habits and had a huge breakfast, lunch and dinner. This was not me—but when I ate, I felt stronger. Now I'm fighting to take it of—even though I went back to my old eating habits, I've only managed to lose about twelve pounds."

Exercise is highly beneficial to chemotherapy patients, but you may not be getting as much as usual. Activity helps burn off calories, curb your appetite, improve your mood, and reduce nausea that you may be trying to alleviate with a steady stream of food. Exercise also takes up the time that you might otherwise fill by eating, as does any distraction. Only four things made me forget about the nausea—food, sleep, exercise, and the movies.

A bloated feeling and appearance can have many causes other than glucocorticoids. Some anticancer drugs can set off processes that render the stomach and intestines less capable of digesting food. Or the digestive process may slow down because of nervousness, tension, a lack of exercise, or constipation. Eating gas-producing foods or swallowing air as you eat can contribute. As a result, the lower abdomen bloats, and you look and feel too full too quickly. Small, frequent meals may help here, as may avoiding hard-to-digest fatty or high-protein foods. Eating slowly and eliminating foods such as onions and cabbage that cause gas may solve the problem. Hydrochloric acid tablets or other digestive aids taken with meals may help reduce the bloated feeling and appearance. Bloating may also be caused by a lactose intolerance. (See pp. 190–91.)

CONSTIPATION

Overall, constipation occurs less frequently in chemotherapy patients than does diarrhea. This condition, which is characterized by infrequent bowel movements, hard, dark, small stools, or straining, is uncomfortable and can be dangerous. The abdomen becomes distended, there is cramping, a decrease in appetite, and possible fecal impaction. Oddly enough, constipation can lead to diarrhea when it increases the bacterial growth within the intestines. The result is explosive diarrhea occurring around the hard stool.

Constipation in chemotherapy patients may be due to a lack of fiber in the diet, the use of narcotics to control pain, a lack of exercise, and emotional stress. Often these are contributing factors to constipation caused by a group of drugs called the vinca alloys: vincristine and vinblastine. Vincristine, for example, has been reported to cause this side effect in 30 percent

of those who get the drug. These drugs are toxic to the nerves.
This leads to a sluggish or paralyzed bowel because the muscle
contractions (peristalsis) that move food through the bowel do
not occur.

Constipation from chemotherapy may occur within twenty-
four hours of treatment, but it may not be obvious until several
courses of treatment have been received. This side effect, when
due to nerve damage, is usually accompanied by numb or
tingling fingers and/or toes. It appears to be minor but is an
early warning of neural drug toxicity, a potentially serious and
nonreversible condition when allowed to progress.

Be sure to tell your physician if you are experiencing constipation. He or she may want to test you to see if there is
nerve damage and adjust your drugs accordingly. Laxatives,
suppositories, enemas, or stool softeners may also be prescribed
as needed, until the condition eases or reverses. Thereafter, or
if the condition is slight, the following measures may help
alone or be used in addition to occasional treatment with the
harsher measures listed above. (The continual use of laxatives
can be habit-forming. They irritate the digestive tract and make
it difficult to have normal bowel movements without them.)

· Eat high-bulk foods: fresh fruit and vegetables—raw or cooked
  but still crisp—dried fruit, whole grain breads and cereals,
  nuts, popcorn, and bran. Add bran to your diet gradually—
  start with two teaspoons a day and slowly work up to two
  tablespoons, then up to four or six. Too much fiber too soon
  can cause cramping, gas, and diarrhea.

· Drink plenty of fluids which the fiber will absorb and keep
  soft.

· Liquid acidophilus, available in health food stores, is another
  natural way to keep "regular."

· Chocolate, coffee, tea, and alcohol tend to stimulate the intestines—but should not be overindulged in.

· Get more exercise—walk, do isometrics.

· Set aside enough "bathroom time" to give sluggish bowels a
  chance to move.

· Take measures to alleviate depression or anxiety. A hot bath
  relaxes you all over—including the sphincter muscle.

DIARRHEA

Diarrhea, to one degree or another, is a common complaint among chemotherapy patients. It occurs when bowel movements are more frequent, loose, and fluid than usual. There is often cramping, flatulence (gas), bloating, and sore, irritated skin around the rectum. Diarrhea is not merely uncomfortable and embarrassing; it can disrupt your life-style and lead to weakness, malnutrition, dehydration, and chemical imbalances because nutrients and water are not properly absorbed by the body.

The anticancer drugs that are the prime culprits in this side effect are the antimetabolites and antibiotics. These drugs kill the rapidly dividing cells that line the intestines. This causes a reduction in the production of the food-digesting enzymes normally present in the intestines, irritation, swelling, and an overproduction of mucus. Neither food nor water is absorbed; and since intestinal activity is stimulated, the food is passed along to the outside world before it is fully digested.

If you suffer from three or more loose bowel movements a day, consult your physician. He or she may suggest that you adopt an all-liquid diet for a few days to give the bowels a rest and then gradually add some low-bulk, "binding" foods. Your doctor may also prescribe anti-diarrhea medication such as Kaopectate or Lomotil.

It is usually advised that the following foods be avoided because they tend to encourage diarrhea—they are either high in fiber or irritate or stimulate the gastrointestinal tract in other ways.

- Whole grain bread and cereal

- Nuts, seeds, coconut, popcorn

- Fried, greasy, fatty foods; pastries, potato chips

- Fresh and dried fruits and fruit juices—exceptions are noted later

- Raw vegetables, cooked vegetables that are gas producing, dried beans and peas

- Strong spices and spicy foods such as chili powder, pepper, curry, garlic, horseradish, olives, pickles, relishes

- Chocolate, alcoholic beverages, coffee, regular tea, tobacco, carbonated beverages (unless they have been allowed to go flat)

- Milk and milk products (also may cause diarrhea—see pp. 190-91)

The following "binding" foods are low in residue or fiber, easily digestible, and tend to be soothing to the digestive tract.

- Soft high-protein foods such as cottage cheese, cream cheese, mild soft cheese, eggs, custards, creamy peanut butter

- Mild high-protein foods such as fish and poultry; low-fat meats such as veal, lamb, some cuts of beef—broiled or roasted rather than fried

- Cooked cereals such as Cream of Wheat, farina

- Some fruits such as bananas (high in potassium), applesauce, peeled apples (contain pectin, an antidiarrheal), apple juice, grape juice, avocados

- White bread or toast

- Macaroni, white rice, noodles; baked, broiled, or mashed potatoes

- Some cooked vegetables such as asparagus tips, green beans, carrots, peas, spinach, squash

- Nutmeg (added to dishes sometimes slows down the digestive tract)

In addition, you should

- Include rest periods during the day if you find you are very tired.

- Drink plenty of fluids to replace the water lost through diarrhea; sip slowly.

- Add foods high in potassium—bananas, apricot and peach nectars, potatoes, broccoli, halibut, asparagus—to replace the potassium depleted during fluid loss. If the problem is severe, your doctor may prescribe a potassium supplement.

· Eat small, frequent meals, slowly—this is easier on the digestive system. Foods served at room temperature or slightly warmer are advised, since very hot or very cold foods can stimulate contractions of the digestive tract.

· Cleanse the rectal area after each bowel movement if it becomes sore from frequent evacuation. Use warm water and a nondrying, nonirritating deodorant-free soap such as Dove, Basis, or castile soap. A healing salve such as Desitine or A & D ointment, or a local anesthetic such as Tucks will give you comfort, as will frequent sitz baths or sitting in a tub of warm water.

MILK INTOLERANCE

Some people are born without the ability to digest milk; a chemotherapy patient, however, may develop this inability because the drugs destroy the cells in the intestine that produce the enzyme (lactase) that digests a milk sugar (lactose). Without lactase, the milk sugar will not be digested, and watery, fermentative diarrhea, flatulence, and cramping result. Since chemotherapy patients often rely heavily on dairy products and add milk-based nutritional supplements to stave off weight loss and malnutrition, this becomes an important symptom to diagnose and treat.

Though there are various laboratory tests that exist to definitively diagnose lactase deficiency, they are not often done because of the time and expense involved. Therefore, the following clues are used: complaints of gas, indigestion, diarrhea, or vague abdominal pain thirty to sixty minutes after drinking milk or eating a milk product.

If you suspect a lactase deficiency, consult your doctor. He or she may recommend that you begin a lactose-free or lactose-reduced diet in addition to adopting the measures suggested in the section on diarrhea.

Patients should cut down or avoid completely foods high in lactose: milk, cream, ice cream, most cheeses, and custard or pudding desserts. Many patients are able to tolerate milk and milk products in which the lactose has been totally or partially broken down: acidophilus milk, lactose-free cottage cheese, yogurt, fermented cheese such as cheddar, and sour cream. In addition, there is a liquid (Lact-aid) that can be added to milk to predigest the lactose.

Many other foods have milk or lactose in their ingredients; read labels carefully. Some of these include: instant coffee, imitation dairy coffee creamers, cocoa and chocolate drinks, breads, party dips, commercial instant potatoes, cakes, cookies, pies, cordials and sherries, sherbert, creamed soups, and chewing gum.

If milk and milk products usually are prominent in your diet as a source of protein, look for foods made with soybean milk. This milk can be bought plain or flavored, in containers just like those with cow's milk, as tofu, which can be substituted for cheese in recipes, and as various forms of "ice cream" deserts. Kosher pareve (milk-free) products can be another good source of protein.

SORE MOUTH, GUMS, AND THROAT

Chemotherapy drugs—particularly the antimetabolites and antibiotics—can produce sores in the mouth (stomatitis), sores in the throat, in the food pipe (esophagitis), and sore, bleeding gums. These side effects are caused by the destruction of fast-growing surface cells in these areas. As a result, minute, raw or bleeding ulcerated patches or spots appear because the blood counts might be low. There may also be a bacterial or fungal infection present, or spontaneous bleeding from the gums. Patients may experience dry mouth, difficulty in chewing and swallowing, an unpleasant taste or odor in the mouth, and alterations in the taste of foods; esophagitis causes mild to severe chest pain which can resemble heartburn.

These side effects can be very painful and distressing and lead to other complications such as loss of weight and malnutrition; gum trouble can lead to a loss of teeth. The soreness usually peaks one week after a treatment and clears up in a few days as the body repairs itself. However, the healing process may be slowed by malnutrition; and deficiencies in zinc, folic acid, riboflavin, and vitamins B_{12} and C can increase the severity.

There is relatively little that can specifically be done to

prevent these side effects from occurring, but there are ways
to alleviate them, minimize them, live with them, and prevent
complications. They *can* be prevented from recurring by reducing the dose of the drug(s) that cause them.

PREVENTIVE DENTISTRY AND ORAL HYGIENE

Starting chemotherapy with a clean, healthy mouth and
maintaining good oral hygiene will go a long way in minimizing
and preventing later mouth problems and infections. Many
oncologists—though not all—advise preventive dentistry for
patients they feel might be at high-risk for oral problems due
to chemotherapy. Dr. William Carl, a dentist at Rosewell Park
Memorial Institute in New York, wrote in an article in the
February 1983 *American Family Physician*:

> "Oral care is very important in patients receiving che-
> motherapy, but it is often overlooked in the urgency of
> a patient's cancer treatment. Ideally, dental evaluation
> and preventive care should become a part of the work-
> up preceding chemotherapy. These measures reduce po-
> tential complications that may be difficult to control later."

Always inform your dentist, preferably before you do it,
that you are undergoing chemotherapy. Although many patients
can safely undergo procedures such as simple fillings and teeth
cleaning while on chemotherapy, it is never certain how any
one patient will react, so it is best to take care of cavities and
rough edges on your teeth before treatment begins. A thorough
cleaning is also advisable because the inevitable minor bleeding
that occurs during cleaning could be serious later on, and because accumulated tartar can harbor bacteria that might infect
mouth sores later on.

If you have gum problems or teeth that are so decayed they
might be abscessed, it is wise to make an appointment with a
dentist and schedule as much work as possible before the treatment begins. Serious procedures such as peridontal surgery or
tooth extraction generally should not be done while you are on
chemotherapy, and the conditions that indicate these procedures
can be worsened by your treatment.

Sometimes chemotherapy can be delayed a few weeks for

this purpose if the likelihood of oral complications from the treatment is great. Your oncologist may be able to recommend a dentist who specializes in the rapid and sometimes radical procedures that are necessary.

If you wear full or partial dentures, it is recommended that you have the fit checked. Have them refit if necessary to avoid irritation and possible infection. Poorly fitting dentures should not be worn; well-fitting ones may be worn after the worst of the side effects of each treatment have subsided. Orthodontic devices (braces) usually are too irritating and need to be removed during chemotherapy.

Floss daily, and clean your mouth after each meal and at bedtime; use a soft-bristled brush and a minimal amount of dentifrice. Rinse afterward with warm saline water (one tablespoon of salt—or one to two tablespoons of baking soda which is milder—in one quart of water). This solution raises the pH of the mouth and helps prevent the growth of acid-loving microorganisms such as candida, which is a yeast infection. Patients are usually advised not to use a commercial mouthwash unless it is alcohol-free, so check the label.

If your blood count is low and stomatitis is severe, avoid dental floss and Water Piks. Clean your teeth gently with a soft-bristled brush or cotton swab. You may be able to find special sponge-tipped swabs (Toothetts) impregnated with a mild dentifrice. After each cleaning, use the following healing, bacteria-fighting rinse which can also be used by itself to clean your teeth if brushing or swabbing is too painful. To make it, mix one part hydrogen peroxide with five parts saline water; add a few drops of alcohol-free mouthwash if desired. Prepare it fresh each time you use it; salt water can be made and kept ahead of time, but the peroxide will lose its effectiveness unless added immediately before using. Swish a mouthful around your mouth for a minute (it will bubble and foam) before spitting it out. Repeat once or twice. You may need to experiment using various proportions and combinations of water, soda, and hydrogen peroxide until you find a rinsing solution you can use frequently without it burning.

MEDICATION AND OTHER MEASURES

Some doctors paint the individual mouth ulcers with an antacid such as milk of magnesia. To do this yourself, use a cotton-tipped swab. Allow the antacid to stand until the liquid rises to the top, pour off the liquid, and dip the swab in the thick white residue. This relieves pain and promotes healing. Antacid simply swished around the mouth will also stick to ulcerations and protect them. If the pain is severe, oncologists sometimes prescribe topical anesthetics such as Xylocaine to kill the pain. These come in spray, lozenge, and liquid forms. If you use such a preparation, be aware of extremely hot foods—you may burn your mouth without realizing it and create further damage.

Dr. William Grace uses viscous lidocaine, a kind of jelly, in his patients with mouth or throat ulcers:

> "This is a kind of Solarcaine for your mouth and is quite good for keeping people's nutritional status up. You may have to swish and swallow a few times to get total anesthesia, and it works only for about twenty minutes to a half hour, but you can get a lot of food down in a half hour. The food doesn't taste like much because lidocaine also numbs the taste buds, but some people learn how to keep it off their tongues so that taste perception is maintained. The other things with stomatitis is that people have a hard time coping with the pain, but pain killers can be given to relieve that."

If an infection is present, your oncologist will prescribe medication: an antibiotic for a bacterial infection, or an anti-fungal for a yeast or fungus infection. Local medication is usually "swished and swallowed"—if the mouth is infected, it is assumed that the esophagus is also.

If your lips become dry and cracked, it is difficult for you to open your mouth wide enough to clean or medicate it. Keep them moist with a soothing cream, drink plenty of liquids, and make sure there is no nutritional deficiency. If you have a history of herpes (cold sores/fever blisters) on the lips, be sure to tell your oncologist who may prescribe an ointment to use to help prevent sores from forming while you are on chemotherapy. If your mouth is very dry, your doctor may prescribe an artificial saliva.

EATING TIPS

- Avoid irritating foods: tart, acidy foods such as citrus fruits and juices, tomatoes, carbonated beverages; hot, spicy foods; and foods that are very dry, coarse, crunchy, or salty and require a lot of chewing and/or saliva to digest such as chips and pretzels, raw vegetables, nuts, and whole grains.

- Avoid tobacco, alcohol, and extremes in temperature—these can injure delicate tissues.

- Nonirritating foods include bland, soft foods such as fruit nectars, creamed soups, soft cheese, eggs, milk shakes, cooked cereals, eggnog, pudding, applesauce, mashed potatoes, and macaroni and cheese. Yogurt may be particularly soothing.

- Try overcooking and puréeing foods such as vegetables and meats to make them easier to eat. Try using junior baby foods. Adding plenty of liquids such as sauces and gravies to foods, or using moist heat in cooking (stewing and steaming) will make food easier to chew and swallow. Have casseroles and soups.

- Drink plenty of fluids—if you are eating less, make nutritious, high-calorie, high-protein drinks. Liquid supplements may be needed to help keep up your nutrient intake. Sipping tepid tea may soothe your mouth and throat.

- Some people find cold foods such as ice cream, ice cubes, frozen yogurt, Popsicles, and sherbert soothing—but others find these things painful.

- If esophagitis is present, milk and milk products such as sour cream, yogurt, and cottage cheese tend to coat the throat and protect the cells. You can eat these every two to four hours.

CHAPTER 12

Hair, Skin, and Nail Effects

The average normal scalp contains 100,000 hairs, 10 to 15 percent of which are in the resting stage at any given time. Most hairs are therefore in the growing stage, which makes them unwitting targets for the effects of many of the most commonly used chemotherapy drugs. In addition to the drugs, a faulty diet and severe stress—particularly from illness, surgery, and emotional trauma—can affect the health of your hair and scalp. The skin and nails can be sensitive to chemotherapy drugs too, although the effects on these are generally more subtle, transitory, and less common than those on the hair.

HAIR LOSS

Chemotherapy patients may lose all or some of the hair on their heads, including the scalp, beard, moustache, eyebrows, and eyelashes. Body hair may eventually thin out or disappear completely—from the arms, armpits, legs, and groin. Though far from dangerous medically, for the patient this loss of hair (alopecia) is often devastating psychologically.

Being bald on top of being sick is a terrible blow to our self-image; it can plunge some of us into the depths of depression or make those who are already depressed even more so. The anxiety about our appearance is a daily insult to our quality of life; it jeopardizes our health and casts doubts upon the wisdom of continuing with chemotherapy. Our hair means so much that sometimes the mere prospect of losing it is enough to make patients refuse to begin a therapy that could save or extend their lives.

Patients' experiences with hair loss and their reactions to it vary greatly. Some say they feel naked, ugly, sexless, and vulnerable, that being bereft of hair is a constant reminder of their cancer. Most do eventually adjust, and a few actually manage to derive pleasure from, or get a few laughs out of, their nearly hairless state:

> "I don't know . . . I had never thought I was vain about my hair. It never really mattered. I had sailed through the surgery and the diagnosis so well, relatively speaking. There I was, traveling through Europe and I had cancer, and I was going through chemotherapy, and I was on top of the world . . . and suddenly, *that* happened to me— and prehistoric feelings of *maleness* were coming out. It was devastating, it really was."

> "Because the drugs took my hair—my scalp hair and moustache too—I become anonymous for two years. All those boring people I didn't have to talk to—I'd just walk right by them in the street. Nobody recognized me. *I* didn't even recognize me. I'd had my beard for ten years and a face can change a lot in that time."

> "You know what? It was a trip being bald. I used to run the pulsating shower over my head!"

I remember being in a yoga class where the teacher came over to me in order to correct my head position. As she touched my head and my wig shifted, she drew back in surprise and said, "Oh your hair!" I looked up with a grin and said, "It isn't mine!"

Edith Imre, the proprietor of Edith Imre Hair Fashions in New York City, who has designed wigs for nearly forty years and has recently devoted much of her own time to fitting cancer patients, thinks that "losing the hair is so devastating because cancer is so often not really visual, and it can be ignored or

denied. But being bald is very visual, a tremendous psychological problem." She tells of one woman, in her thirties, who
came into her salon. "She was completely beyond herself,
saying, 'I want to die, I want to die.'" Another businesswoman
client of hers found the hair loss a greater blow than the cancer;
she quit her job and refused to talk to friends. An elderly
gentleman felt like a freak; he became a recluse because he
feared ridicule.

One oncology nurse supervisor remarked, "among side effects, hair loss is the one that patients are the most disturbed
about. That's what you present to the public; it's the first thing
others see. I had had patients who refused chemotherapy because they didn't want to lose their hair."

It is important for chemotherapy patients to know that not
all drugs cause hair loss. And those that are known for this
side effect do not always cause it in every individual or to the
same extent.

Fifteen percent of chemo patients do not lose their hair.
Except in very rare cases, hair loss from chemotherapy is temporary. The hair does grow back after the chemotherapy is
stopped, and sometimes before that if the hair growth becomes
resistant to the drugs. Although losing your hair is traumatic,
embarrassing, and terribly inconvenient, there are psychological and practical ways to prepare yourself and to cope with
the possibility or actuality.

MINIMIZING THE EFFECTS

Many patients want to know if there are ways they can make
the possibility or reality of losing their hair less traumatic psychologically; whether they can make their hair look better if it
becomes thinner from chemotherapy; if there is anything they
can do to prevent, delay, or minimize their hair loss.

The first step in coping with this side effect is to get an idea
of what you will be dealing with. Be sure to talk over your
concerns with your doctor. Ask how likely it is that the drugs
you will be taking will cause hair loss, how much you can
expect to lose, and when. Although in most cases it is impossible to be very specific or sure, in others the track record is
clear. At any rate, for many patients the experience of losing
their hair is harder if their doctor downplays the possibility,

extent, or importance. Ms. Imre asserts that "Doctors can be so stupid and insensitive. One woman told me that her doctor said, 'Look at me—I'm bald too. So what's the big deal?'"

Mr. Nicholas, the wig stylist for the Kenneth Beauty Salon in New York, comments:

> "People who are unprepared take the bad road. I get asked a lot of questions about what I've seen or what they should expect because most of the doctors don't give their patients enough information. Some do care and understand that this is one of the major problems that people face when they go through chemotherapy. Some doctors are right up front—they tell patients they might lose their hair—either because that's the way they are, or because with some types of therapies they can be more sure than with others."

Donna Park says:

> "It's fine for doctors to say that chemotherapy causes hair loss. But you really need to get down to the nitty-gritty. Which drugs do; which drugs don't; which ones do to a certain degree. For instance, 90 percent of the patients who receive Adriamycin do lose their hair. But you're not going to wake up the morning after your first treatment and find all your hair on your pillow. One patient I know had overheard other women talking about wigs. She became very frightened and asked, 'Where am I going to find a wig tonight?' I had to tell her she wouldn't wake up bald the next morning, but that she should start looking for a wig."

When my hair fell out, I was devastated. I can't deny that vanity played its part, but a good deal of the blame lies in my not being well enough prepared. My oncologist did warn me that it all might fall out, but said it was possible that only some of it might. He observed that since I had a lot of hair to begin with, I could afford to lose some. He mentioned that a lot of people on chemo get wigs, but I said, "Not me! Even if some hair falls out, I'm not so vain that I can't live with hair that looks a little thin." I thought I'd wait and see if I needed one. I don't know if he was soft-pedaling hair loss in order to be kind and not to scare me off, or if it just didn't sink in that I might become totally bald and what this would mean to me. As a result, I was total unprepared—in psychological and practical terms—when it did fall out, all of it.

The incidence of scalp hair loss varies from individual to individual and depends in part upon the drug dosage. Nevertheless, some drugs have a higher potential to cause this than others have. In "Alopecia and Chemotherapy," an article published in the May 1980 issue of *The American Journal of Nursing*, the drugs listed as being the most common causes of alopecia were: cyclophosphamide (Cytoxan), doxorubicin (Adriamycin), and vincristine (Oncovin); moderately common were actinomycin-D (Cosmegen), bleomycin, daunorubicin, and Methotrexate.

As a general rule, hair begins to fall out within three or four treatments. It may begin sooner and peak one or two months afterward. In some people, it falls out very gradually or the loss is so slight it is hardly noticeable. In others it falls out in huge clumps or all at once. Some people wear caps or scarves to bed to catch the shedding hair. People can become completely bald except for a slight "peach fuzz" effect. If the hair doesn't all fall out but becomes thinner, it can continue to grow, but with a change in texture and appearance.

"I woke up one morning, lifted my head up, and my hair just stayed there, on the pillow."

"My hair had been falling out a little bit. I lathered up my head, began to massage my scalp, and with a sinking feeling I could almost feel the whole thing shift . . . with the water and the lather . . . I got almost physically sick. I know I at least came close to tears; I don't think I actually cried. But I was paralyzed. I couldn't do anything. I just felt disgusting with all this hair all over the place. My wife came in and had to finish rinsing me off and cleaning out the tub while I got out and tried to not throw up. It was really devastating."

"I lost a lot of my hair—but not all of it. I'd say I've lost half of it. I don't need a wig; I've always had a lot of hair. Now it just looks sparse—people come up to me and say it looks gorgeous—I used to have too much hair. I wear it very close-cropped and I trim it every three weeks. The texture has changed—I used to have very curly hair and now it's straight. And it breaks. It still looks good, but it's not me."

The onset of my hair loss was much more difficult to deal with than it had to be because as I said earlier, I was so ill-prepared; my being away from home when it happened made it even more of a nightmare. I had had three treatments and I didn't feel too bad at all. No hair had fallen out so I figured I was home free and would be spared the worst of the side effects. Full of relief and nonchalance, I went on a trip. In a glorious example of "perfect" timing, my hair began to shed slightly on the plane. Four days later, I was barely presentable: You could see right through to my scalp. There I was stuck, away from home with no scarf, no wig, in unfamiliar surroundings with nowhere to hide. I finally found a few horrendous scarves to wear, which at least left me looking human. I cried a lot during that week; I never felt so down at any other time because finally toxicity had built up. Not only had my hair fallen out, but I was beginning to feel physically ill because of the nausea and tiredness that had hit at the same time. Eventually, I bought a wig that looked fine, but I still felt a sense of revulsion every time I saw myself without it. Losing my hair was the most dramatic, tangible side effect I experienced. Everything else was vague and invisible, or purely medical. Then I not only felt sick, I looked sick.

If your oncologist seems unable to help you cope, speaking with a counselor such as a nurse or social worker, or with a patient who has had or is having chemotherapy may help you to prepare yourself psychologically for hair loss. All the sources for emotional support discussed in Chapter 6 will help you adjust both to possible and actual loss of hair.

Most experienced professionals recommend that patients begin to look for a wig, and possibly buy one, before beginning chemotherapy and before the hair has started to fall out. Although many patients may not need or want a wig, many others will; and the peace of mind in knowing that an attractive hairpiece is handy is an important factor in how well people cope with hair loss. Donna Park says the advantage to looking for a wig early is "So that when you start to feel uncomfortable—either from the other side effects or because the hair loss is noticeable—you're not pressured to go out and buy something that you really can't afford or one that isn't right for you. You need time to shop around to find something that's right." Or, some other kind of head covering should be on hand—turbans, scarves, hats, and caps are preferred by some instead of wigs, or are used until they obtain a wig.

Because hair loss is one of the more distressing side effects, numerous attempts have been made to prevent it. Recently, some patients have been able to prevent some scalp hair loss through the use of tourniquets or ice-filled caps. These devices are placed on the head during chemotherapy treatments in an effort to reduce the flow of blood there, and hence, expose the hair follicles in the scalp to lower concentrations of the drugs. Techniques vary, but generally when a tourniquet is used, it is worn during and immediately after the injection and is left on for up to twenty or forty-five minutes afterward. When ice is used, it is put on five minutes before and left on for about fifteen minutes after the injection.

This practice is not the answer to all chemotherapy patients' prayers, however. While it has met with some success, the effectiveness varies greatly and total prevention of hair loss is not yet possible. The ice and tourniquets are uncomfortable. People report headaches, chills, and dizziness from them. When drugs are given by slow infusion, or oral chemotherapy is taken several times a day, the devices would have to be left on too long to be safe or comfortable for the patient.

Many physicians do not endorse the use of the tourniquets or caps except under certain conditions. They feel this practice should be avoided in patients for whom chemotherapy offers a chance for a cure, because there is the danger of creating a sanctuary for tumor cells circulating in the scalp. This is the case in adjuvant chemotherapy and in some metastatic diseases that can be cured, as well as with leukemias and lymphomas, where the chemotherapeutic intent is to kill every single malignant cell.

Dr. William Grace, an oncologist in New York's St. Vincent's Hospital, says:

"The problem with chemo caps in the propensity to develop scalp relapses in people who are being treated for a cure. This is not theoretical—I've seen it and it has been confirmed several times in the literature. I had a patient whose disease went into remission everywhere but the scalp line—where it grew."

Patients are usually responsible for bringing their own tourniquets or caps and for obtaining and maintaining ice—no mean task when the wait for your treatment can stretch to hours. Donna Park says the patient has to get a written order from the physician and the policy varies from physician to physician at Memorial.

"Because of the controversy, the decision is left up to the patient and the physician. If the patients want ice caps they have to bring in their own. We'll put them in the refrigerator; but if something has to remain frozen, patients come in with ice chests."

Some people try to hold onto their hair once it starts falling out. Often, they stop shampooing it or combing it because they have heard that this will keep it in longer. Black people, whose hair can be tightly braided and left untouched, have some success with this approach. The hairs that don't come loose from the scalp anchor the ones that do; this and the texture helps maintain the illusion of a full head of hair.

For those with smooth textured hair, the "don't touch" approach doesn't really work well. Mr. Nicholas has had clients who have tried it:

"Once it starts falling out, it's going to come out. But if you don't touch it—if you don't pull it, wash it, or comb it—it's gong to stay in longer—if you can handle it. Some people do; some are nervous, frightened, and sensitive and don't want any of their hair to come out until their wig is ready. I've seen people who haven't touched their hair for four weeks. But their hair is uncomfortable and it doesn't look good—it is dirty, dull, matted. I will cut off the matted hair when they are ready for it. I do think it is much more comfortable for them if they got the shortest possible haircut that they will be comfortable with. It's a lot less dramatic or traumatic when it's short and close than when it's long and becoming matted. It's a lot easier to deal with thinning hair when it's short."

Many others recommend that patients cut their hair short before it starts falling out. Joseph Rodriguez, general manager of the Vidal Sassoon Salon in New York, has had many clients who have undergone chemotherapy:

"Clients come in, they tell me that they are beginning chemotherapy and that their doctors recommend that they get a haircut. I always suggest that we cut the hair very short—as short as possible—as long as it suits them. It will be easier for them and make the hair last longer. When the hair is short, it looks thicker. Shorter hair keeps the hair strong because you don't pull it when you comb it, so it is easy to manage. And when it falls out, there will not be the additional problem of matting hair."

I, for one, can vouch for the advisability of taking this step. My doctor recommended getting a haircut before my hair started falling out but didn't say how short. I just lopped four inches of my shoulder-length hair—why give up more than I had to? I thought maybe it wouldn't fall out after all. If I knew then what I know now! About half of it came loose during one shampooing. I could feel it matting as I lathered up. I ended up with instant dreadlocks that wouldn't budge. Losing so much hair at once was a bad enough shock, but now I had a gargantuan task ahead of me, and I thought I would never be able to untangle that rat's nest. Using an Afro pick, crying and feeling sick to my stomach, I pulled and tugged for an hour and cursed the fact that the pulling was making even more hair fall out. If I had gotten a much shorter haircut it definitely wouldn't have been as bad an experience.

Often the hair growth is not completely halted, and some hair remains. Chemotherapy can sometimes just shrink the hair bulb, or root, which constricts the hair shaft as it grows. The hair—chemo hair—becomes thinner, sparser, weaker, of a brittle, finer texture, and takes on a dull appearance. Those with thick, strong, bouncy, curly hair find themselves with limp, straight hair. These people usually do not wear wigs and are still "presentable" but can be far from happy with their appearance:

"My hair didn't fall out completely, but it was a mess. It was very thin and fine; it was always shiny and now it was drab. I looked like a nun who had just come out of the convent. I'd turn my head and hair would fall out—there was hair over everything. I went to my hairdresser and he asked me, 'What have you done?' I burst into tears and told him I hadn't done anything, that I was on chemo. We tried henna, everything, to thicken and liven it up, but nothing worked."

"I never got a wig, though I played with the idea because my hair had gotten very thin; it was straight, with no life, and it just lay there. I'd show pictures of myself to people I had just met, who didn't know me before the chemo, and say, 'This isn't me—this picture is the real me.' I wore a lot of hats—I love them—I had different hats for different outfits."

To look its best, chemo hair should be treated gently, shampooed often, and styled to make the most of what's there. Avoid harsh hard-bristled brushes, sleeping with hair rollers, chemical treatments such as coloring or permanents, and hot hair dryers. The so-called hair thickeners are not recommended because they leave only a temporary coating along each hair shaft, they give the hair the appearance of thickness but leave a gummy deposit which dulls the hair further. As Mr. Rodriguez says:

"Thickeners do not work. If they did, I would use them on my hair, which is very fine and thin. Let's face it: There is not a whole lot you can do for a person whose hair is falling out. I think the best thing is to get a good short haircut and keep the scalp clean. If the hair falls out heavily, there is nothing you can do but wear a scarf, hat, or wig."

In our culture it is much more acceptable for men than for women to be bald. Generally women feel much more uncomfortable without their hair than do men. Hereditary baldness, far more common among men, has occurred in male role models—fathers, grandfathers, entertainment personalities, and great men of history. Too, stunning female "Star Trek" aliens notwithstanding, bald men are considered still normal, masculine, and sometimes even sexy. Many men on chemotherapy shave their heads rather than see their hair fall out before their very eyes, or walk around with a head of thinning hair, or suffer the expense, discomfort, and inconvenience of wearing a hairpiece. Bald is just their "new look." However, many others do cling to whatever is left and are deeply affected by hair loss.

BUYING A WIG OR HAIRPIECE

Having a wig in which you feel comfortable is an important factor in the difficult process of coping with hair loss. After having been fitted with wigs, Edith Imre's clients have told her that keeping their spirits up is an important part of the treatment; then they feel "hopeful, relieved, not like outcasts." "At least now I can leave the house without a hat, or feeling that I'm going to scare the kiddies in the neighborhood," said one. "You don't know what a feeling of comfort and confidence this is to me," said another.

Mr. Nicholas says, "The better people look, the better they adjust to baldness. If you have a lousy wig on, you'll feel terrible. Many patients see others wearing bad wigs in the doctor's office and they are turned off by them."

Wigs are available through barbers, hairdressers, beauty salons, wig specialty shops, from wig suppliers directly, through the mail, and in department stores. They may be made of real or synthetic hair, prestyled, ready-made (the equivalent of "off the rack"), handmade or custom-made. The kind of wig or hairpiece you get and where you buy it depends upon your individual taste, how important it is for you to duplicate your own hair, how much money you can spend, where you live, what's available, and how much time you have.

For me, buying a wig was a relatively simple matter in which luck played a big part. I just looked up "Wigs" in the yellow pages and made a few phone calls: I knew I didn't want to spend much. I went to a wig supplier—real primitive conditions. I looked at the samples, picked out a couple, hid in the bathroom to try them on, and that was that. I was lucky—I paid only forty dollars for the one I ended up with, and it was a mass of natural looking curls very close to my own hair color but very different from my usual style. So I didn't have to worry about a phony looking part or hairline, or explaining everything to people I only knew sightly. It was the right style, and perfect strangers would walk up to me on the street and ask where I got my perm. I'd send them to my hairdresser of course.

You would do best, though, if you allow yourself as much time as possible for the selection, ordering, and preparation of your hairpiece. You can begin by asking your oncologist, nurse, or social worker to recommend a source for a good wig—they have probably seen many different hairpieces and are in a good position to judge. Or you can ask a fellow patient who you know is wearing one that you like.

To feel most comfortable and look most natural, wigs should be fitted and styled professionally. If you get the names of several sources, you can shop around and compare. Most of the preliminary scouting can be done over the phone—find out about the types of wigs available, the price range, the waiting time, the personality of the wig stylist, and the degree of privacy.

It is advisable for chemotherapy patients to buy their wigs before their hair falls out, and many do; however, many do not. Therefore, for many people, the last two factors—the stylist's personality and the degree of privacy—are very important and should not be overlooked. As one patient said, "When you lose your hair, your spirits fall and you are ashamed to be seen. A regular salon is inappropriate for a chemo patient who is not buying a wig for fun and pleasure, and who doesn't want to explain or show hair loss to a stranger."

More than enough has been said or written about the psychotherapeutic overtones in the client-hairdresser relationship. Suffice it to say that this aspect can assume even more importance when the client is a cancer patient who has lost his or her hair. One of Ms. Imre's patients told her, "You saw the pain inside me and used patience and understanding to help tremendously." Out of a desire to help people who could not afford wigs, Ms. Imre has established a foundation called the Institute for Loss of Hair and has given away over six thousand wigs to hospitals and the American Cancer Society. She says, "Nothing gives me more pleasure than to see the feeling of joy in the faces of unfortunate and suffering human beings."

Mr. Nicholas also stresses the importance of understanding and patience for his special clients:

> "You develop a more personal relationship with clients that are going to have chemotherapy than you do with people who are just coming in for haircuts. They have to rely on you a little bit more and you have to understand what they're going through and be able to deal with it. Because they are not always going to feel well, they're

not always easy to get along with. They can get difficult, and it can be frustrating, but that's part of being in this business. When people are having problems, you have to be understanding."

In wigs synthetic hair is less expensive than human hair both in terms of initial cost and upkeep. Synthetic wigs are easy to maintain since they do not require "setting." Some look unnatural, but natural looking ones can be found. Human hair wigs generally look more natural. However, they are more expensive and require more care than synthetic wigs. Both kinds have a mesh or lace base, which varies in degree of give, comfort, appearance, and practicality. Wig prices range from a thirty-dollar ready-made synthetic to a fifteen hundred- or two thousand-dollar handmade human hair wig that will match your own hair perfectly. Higher quality synthetic wigs cost a few hundred dollars and up.

Most experts agree with Ms. Imre who believes:

"It's very important that a wig be easy to handle. I wouldn't recommend human hair wigs—they're too expensive, too delicate, and require too much care. Especially if someone isn't feeling well most of the time, he or she doesn't want to be bothered with taking care of a wig. It should be comfortable, and the base should not be made of a very large mesh—this is okay for someone who still has some hair, but in a totally bald person, the bare scalp will show through."

"There are really two types of people," Ms. Imre says. "Those who want to look as much as possible like they did before, and those who go in the opposite direction." Most people still have at least some of their hair when they come to a salon for a wig. If they don't, the stylist asks them to bring in a photograph or has them describe how they looked.

Mr. Nicholas feels it can be difficult for people to find a natural looking wig:

"Ready-made, prestyled synthetic wigs tend to look very artificial unless you are very lucky. This type of wig can be helped if your hairdresser styles it. Ready-made is the least expensive and faster to buy. When I start off with one of these, I take a sample of the person's hair and buy the wig that's closest in color and texture to it. I then fit, cut, and style it on the person's head. This I can do in a week or less, depending upon the availability of a matching wig."

Handmade and custom-made stretch wigs look better, are more comfortable and lighter on the head, and less hot in the summer. They are much more expensive (up to two thousand dollars at Kenneth) and there's a longer wait (up to six weeks) for them to be ready. Nevertheless, people do order them, and some come from all over the country and the world to have their wigs made at Kenneth. (Real hair wigs can be made from your own hair, provided it is cut off early—once it falls out it is too tangled to use.)

If possible, you should buy the wig in person. Only then can you be assured of getting the best fit and most flattering style. Some recommend bringing a friend along, but Ms. Imre feels differently:

"Bring a spouse instead. A friend or sister comes in with a chemotherapy patient who doesn't have any hair and it's very difficult. The friend starts in, 'Oh she had such beautiful hair, you should have seen how thick it was.' I tell you, this only makes the woman feel worse. Don't people realize how damaging this is?"

With the proper care, a good wig can last up to a year of moderate wear, so many recommend that you buy two wigs. You might want one that resembles your own hair and another that's very different, just for fun. Mr. Nicholas advises that "people have a good one, that's comfortable and always looks good, and a cheaper one that they can wear when their good wig is being serviced, or for everyday, or for times like emptying the garbage. Usually two wigs will do it for a year."

Some people become so devastated and self-conscious about their appearance that they remove their wigs only for sleeping and showering. However, wigs can be pretty uncomfortable, especially after weeks of daily wear. Many people, though shy at first, eventually loosen up, give way to comfort, and do not wear their hairpieces at all times. Most children and spouses quickly adjust to the appearance of the chemotherapy patient, and, of course, do not love them any less because they are temporarily bald. Families understand that at a time when you are not feeling well, every little bit of understanding helps. It is a show of trust and security to let those close to you see you as you really are. As one woman said to me, "I run around a lot without my hairpiece because it's so hot and uncomfortable. My kids are used to it; they don't care—I'm still Mom."

I liked the way my wig looked, but sometimes I hated the way it felt. As is the case with my shoes it was a relief to be rid of the wig and I couldn't wait to take it off the minute I got home. I was very self-conscious about it, though Michael, god bless him, tried to convince me he actually preferred me bald. I felt so naked, so vulnerable, so ugly. We tried to make jokes about this and he gave me the nickname "Baldielocks." At times he'd make me feel better about it by cradling my head in his hands and gently stroking my peach fuzz. Still, I often wore a scarf or knitted cap instead of the wig, although this was partly because my head got surprisingly cold without the protection of my usual mane of long blonde hair.

Turbans can alternately or completely take the place of a full wig. They come in many colors and are stretchy, soft, and comfortable. A turban stays on easily and stands up to wear and tear, so it is especially useful on days you feel really sick or during a treatment cycle if you are a hospital inpatient. The somewhat severe look of a turban can be softened with a small wiglet attached to the front so that some hair peeks out from underneath. This combination is more comfortable than a wig, less expensive, and more practical, and still gives the illusion of hair.

Hairpieces needed as a result of medical treatment are a tax deductible expense, and some insurance policies cover them. Wigs can be obtained free—or their cost defrayed—through the social service departments of some hospitals and clinics, the American Cancer Society, and other agencies, organizations, and foundations. Wigs can also be obtained through public assistance programs.

FACIAL AND BODY HAIR

Although most patients find the loss of scalp hair the most distressing, some find the loss of facial or body hair just as disturbing, if not more. Donna Park remarks that some patients say that losing the hair on their heads was more acceptable

than losing the hair on other parts of their bodies. And people
don't realize they can lose their pubic hair. "I had one woman
who said she felt like "a plucked chicken." I found it weird,
but not unpleasant, to be as hairless as a nine-year-old again,
and not to have to shave my legs or underarms for months was
a definite plus.

There is not much you can do about replacing or disguising
the loss of facial or body hair. You can wear eyebrow and
eyelash makeup, or eyeglasses with large frames and tinted
lenses. Mr. Nicholas says he suggests that if a woman's hair-
style can cover her brow line, she can leave it a little bit longer
than usual. False eyebrows, eyelashes, moustaches, and beards
do exist, but people rarely ask for them.

WHEN THE HAIR GROWS BACK

The loss of hair brought about by chemotherapy is almost
always reversible. Regrowth often begins even before the treatment is over, as the hair grows resistant to the chemicals. This
initial growth may appear to be abnormal: People with straight
hair commonly grow curly hair—to the surprise of many patients. It may at first, however, be finer, or silkier, or of a
different color or texture. This chemo hair is a transient stage;
the hair eventually becomes thicker—in many cases thicker
than before the therapy—and usually eventually returns either
completely back to normal or nearly so.

I spoke with this patient six months after he had completed
his chemotherapy and was due for a second haircut; he said of
his hair: "It feels a little softer and is curly. My barber says it
feels like infant's hair. If I just step out of the shower and don't
comb it, it's a mass of Byronic curls. In fact, I'm thinking of
going as Byron to a costume party next month. It's definitely
less gray than it was, but my beard is more gray."

Once the hair starts growing back, when and how to "come
out" can be an agonizing decision; it can be a difficult transitional period. Some people are ecstatic when their hair re-
grows and they discard their wigs at the earliest possible moment.
I was elated when my hair began to grow back three months
after it had fallen out—I felt the stubble, or as my oncologist
called it, the "five o'clock shadow." I kept rubbing my head
in glee and disbelief. Nevertheless, I had to wait another three
months until I could appear in public without a wig, my hair
was so thin and fine. Still, it was only a half-inch long when

I began to seriously entertain thoughts of appearing au naturel. I did it in stages: first, I took out the garbage, just to see how it felt to be outdoors. It felt okay! Then I mailed a letter in the mailbox across the street. No one stared: no one ran away screaming! Then, getting braver by the minute, I went to the grocery store and made actual contact with people. Still no reaction. That was it from then on. I hadn't trusted my friends who said: "Do it, do it," or Michael who said "Well, it *is* awfully short." I had to test it out myself.

Others are reluctant to give up their wigs because they prefer the way they look over their real hair. A social worker told me about a patient who began shaving her head when her hair started to grow back because it was uncomfortable under a wig, which she wanted to continue to wear. Mr. Nicholas says:

> "Half the people can't wait to throw out their wigs and stomp on them when their hair has grown back. The other half have learned to like their wigs, especially if they're expensive ones. They get compliments when they wear their wigs and use them when their hair isn't right. Usually they buy new hairpieces, though, because their chemotherapy wigs are usually pretty worn out by then."

He also tells of the problem faced by patients who have been coloring the hair blond before the chemotherapy, and whose hair grows back gray mixed with brown and sticks out from under their blond wigs. "I tell these people to check with their doctors, and if it's okay, we'll lighten up just around the hairline so it can be combed in with the wig." Ms. Imre says patients often use water-soluble rinses to cover hair that is growing in gray, because of the cancer scare with stronger dyes, which may also be too harsh for the new growth.

Some people can't wait to run out and get perms to make their new hair look better. This, as is true with hair coloring, is usually not advisable unless the hair is strong and has a good texture—check with your doctor. What is advisable is a haircut as soon as there is hair to cut. "Once hair starts growing in and looking straggly," says Mr. Nicholas, "I like to have my clients come in and I'll trim it—clean it up. That makes people feel comfortable about themselves. They can look better with their own hair, and pretty soon they'll be wearing their wigs only for special occasions."

SKIN CHANGES

The skin can be affected by chemotherapy in many ways. Most effects are minor and disappear between treatments or after the course of therapy is over. Some patients experience dry, itchy, flaky, sensitive skin while on chemotherapy. The reason for this is since the skin cells multiply rapidly, the skin sheds more than usual and becomes thin. The sweat glands may also be affected, which leaves the skin drier than usual, as one patient describes. A breast cancer patient recalls:

"I was concerned that my skin was going to get old fast from the chemo. I didn't get wrinkles or creases, but my skin did get very dry. I looked like I had dandruff all over my body—not just my head. When I peeled off my stockings I'd shake them out and flakes of skin would fall. It was disgusting! I used *a lot* of Nivea. And when my scalp got dry I used mineral oil on it, and baby oil, but that just made my thin hair look limper and thinner."

Patients with problem skin should protect it from harsh, cold, dry weather and too much water. Long hot baths tend to dry skin even further; quick showers and sponge baths with super-fatted nondrying soaps are better. Daily use of emollient and moisturing creams and lotions is recommended; used immediately after washing while the skin is still damp, they help seal in moisture. Raising the humidity in the house with a humidifier will also help.

If your scalp becomes itchy and flaky, a dandruff shampoo may help, as may oil rubbed into the scalp, although as mentioned above, this can make thinning hair look worse. Wearing a wig or head covering has not been shown to affect hair growth, but it can increase perspiration, dandruff, and itching and can irritate a sensitive, newly bared scalp. Frequent cleansing with a mild shampoo and keeping the head uncovered whenever possible will help here.

The skin may be prone to more bacterial and fungal infections than usual because of its increased sensitivity and a person's lowered resistance to disease in general. These local infections should be treated with local medication; refer to Chapter 10 for information about protecting the immune system and avoiding infections.

Some drugs cause changes in skin color, and these may be triggered or worsened by exposure to sunlight. Many patients are advised to avoid the sun, although others are permitted to sunbathe in moderation. Check with your doctor to see if your drugs can cause photosensitivity; if they do, wear protective clothing, hats, and a sun block while in the sun. The areas usually affected by the drug-sun combination are the backs of the hands, bodily creases, nails and nail beds, the face, and the elbows. Rarely, the skin over the whole body can be affected.

Some drugs can cause a local irritation or red rash around the injection site. This is not serious and should disappear within an hour or two after the treatment. Some drugs may also cause the veins to darken. This is not serious either, and the vein is not damaged; the darkness should disappear within a week or two. Patients may also experience mild discomfort during an injection, both from the needle and the drugs themselves. This should not be confused with *extravasation*, a potentially serious complication that occurs at the site of the injection when some of the drug escapes into the surrounding tissue, rather than into the vein where it belongs. This is a slight, though real, danger with intravenous therapy.

There are varying degrees of extravasation; even though my oncologist was very careful, I had a minor brush with it myself. I usually avoided looking at the injection site during a treatment, but I couldn't help but take a peek the time I felt more pain than usual. I saw a mound of purple swelling in the crook of my arm, but I wasn't really worried—yet. My oncologist told me the mound was blood mixed with vincristine. I made some jokes about whether this was how people got those special effects in the movies; he patched me up and continued the injection in another vein. The pain became so bad I hardly slept that night, and when I called him he prescribed a very strong cortisone cream. In a few hours, it felt much better and the swelling went way down. I put ice on it all week, and when the time for my next shot rolled around, two weeks later, it was almost completed healed.

Most, but not all, drugs cause problems if they leak into the surrounding tissue. Methotrexate, for example, is harmless—it can be injected into the muscle. But extra precautions should always be taken with a drug such as Adriamycin, which is perhaps the most caustic anticancer drug. Dangerous drugs that can cause *necrosis* (tissue death) should not be the first or the last substances to enter the vein; they should be safely sandwiched between either harmless drugs or a saline solution. After the treatment is over and the needle is withdrawn, rather than applying pressure with the arm in the usual lowered bent elbow position, some doctors have their patients raise their arms up over their heads as they apply pressure to the injection site. This collapses the vein nicely and prevents any remains of the drugs from backing up out of the vein and causing problems.

The sooner extravasation is caught, the better. Always tell the doctor or nurse of any pain or burning sensation during the injection so they can check whether the reaction is normal or if something is amiss. Try to keep movement to a minimum during treatment, and complain like hell if you are being treated by a clumsy technician.

Another danger with intravenous chemotherapy is "blown" veins. Preferred veins, those used again and again during blood tests and chemotherapy, get a real workout. Eventually, they may say "enough" by shutting down in protest, becoming hard, and no longer allowing the blood to flow through. This is not particularly dangerous since other blood vessels will learn to take over, but it may make treatment gradually more and more difficult as more and more "good veins" get used up.

Occasionally, phlebitis may occur. This is a painful inflammation of the vein that is somewhat common in patients taking drugs they are sensitive to. Treatment for phlebitis includes application of heat and oral painkillers. This condition takes several weeks to subside.

NAIL PROBLEMS

Discolored and disfigured nails are a rare complication of chemotherapy. Nails can become brittle, cracked, and ridged; they may tear, flake, and break off painfully near the quick. Remedies for hardening and strengthening brittle nails have not been proven, but they are generally harmless and, unless you experience a reaction to the ingredients, may help. Nail polish—especially the kinds containing nylon fibers—can support and protect the nail; use as many coats as necessary to form a thick enough shield. You can minimize the dangers and damage to your nails by wearing rubber gloves and protective gloves when performing chores; using rich hand creams may also help if you massage around the nail beds with them.

CHAPTER 13

Effects on Sexuality

Many patients are eager to know about how chemotherapy affects people's sex lives. As Grace Christ of New York's Memorial Sloan-Kettering says, "Sexuality is a product of many things. Chemotherapies do impact on sexuality—but we're not sure as to how." Some patients report an increase in sexual activity; others say there is no difference. Many, however, do report a decrease to varying degrees:

> "I would say there's moderate sex on chemo. We weren't exactly swinging from the chandeliers . . . but I did feel like 'doing it.' I did feel somewhat asexual because of the combination of a lost breast and the lost hair. I couldn't imagine how anybody would want me."

> "Sex? There is no sex on chemo. My husband and I sat down and talked about it and he really understood. We always had a really nice sexual relationship, and suddenly I had no interest whatsoever. It wasn't because of the mastectomy; it had nothing to do with my feeling less desirable. I was just indifferent. Fortunately, we learned to live with it; we knew it was temporary."

Obviously side effects due to chemo such as tiredness, infection, nausea, weight fluctuations, hair loss, depression, low

216

self-esteem, and fear of losing a partner can lower our libidos and inhibit us sexually. Chemotherapy may also affect hormone levels and otherwise throw our reproductive systems off course.

As with other side effects, there are no hard and fast rules. Science has taught us that the brain is the most potent sexual organ there is: The mind is the true source of our sexuality. Our mental attitude can be a surprisingly powerful force both in overcoming any obstacles that chemo has placed in our path, and in adapting to those it cannot override. Though sexual intercourse may be put on the back burner, many people have found that sexual expression is not. Sex during chemotherapy may not be quite the same as before, but it can still be enjoyable and satisfying for both partners.

If sexuality is important to you (and to many people it is not, at least at this time), and you find yours is being adversely affected, help can be found through many channels. As one of the patients just quoted has shown us, having honest, open discussions with your partner is an excellent place to start, and may be all you need. In addition, you might seek out medical solutions or outside psychological support, or brush up on your sex education and learn about alternatives to previous sexual habits and preferences. Remember, it is natural to have some concerns and questions about sexuality in relation to cancer treatment, although this issue is not often discussed openly with patients and very little information is volunteered. You may even find that your questions are being avoided, but don't allow this to convince you that your fears and thoughts are imaginary or foolish. Don't give up if sexual satisfaction and expression rank high in your needs and their absence or diminishment poses a threat to your quality of life.

YOU AND YOUR PARTNER

The keys to enjoyable sexual activity for anyone are the ability to communicate openly, to relax, and to be flexible. This is no less true for people who are having chemotherapy. The quality of the relationship, the sexual skills, and the affection between partners that existed previously also help to determine the level of sexual enjoyment during chemo.

If chemo does impose changes in the way you're feeling emotionally and physically, you must make your new needs and limitations known. For example, you may be ready to resume sexual activity but your partner may not realize it; or sex may be the furthest thing from your mind, but not your partner's. You might want to be sociable or affectionate at this time, but not sexual.

Psychological and emotional factors may cause us to withdraw from the whole experience, as a way of protecting ourselves from possible failure or rejection. Whether we try to express our sexuality or we withdraw depends also, to a large extent, on our sexual partners, be they permanent (a spouse or constant lover) or randomly available. Although rejection is a real possibility—partners may find chemo patients unattractive, or fear catching the disease, or be afraid of hurting them, or be reluctant to bother them "after all they've been through"—these anxieties are often not grounded in reality.

Often, whatever differences happen because of chemo, they are fortunately short-lived. If you had a good relationship and enjoyed sexual activity before your illness, chances are these things will reassert themselves eventually of their own accord. Sometimes the increased closeness that a serious illness can bring between two people will not only change their sexual relationship, it will ultimately change it for the better.

There's more to sex, love, and affection than intercourse and/or orgasms. Even when you are too ill or tired, or when surgery is too recent for you to indulge in the athletics of the whole sexual gamut, you and your partner can express yourselves sexually—and have a very good time doing it. As adults, we have come to think of kissing, cuddling, and caressing as preludes, but they are quite nice all by themselves.

In my household, sex wasn't exactly a thing of the past, but it sure wasn't what it used to be. We often found ourselves content with the less vigorous forms of affection and appreciation. That was what I needed most at the time, not more excitement! The simply fact of having a warm, caring body next to mine was immensely reassuring, comforting, therapeutic, and meaningful. Gentle, heartfelt, loving stroking and hugging were good for my body and the soul; they helped heal me emotionally and increased my sense of physical well-being too.

And just as you can have intercourse without orgasm, you can have orgasms without intercourse. As Kinsey and Masters and Johnson have shown, the parameters of healthy sexual behavior are broader than we thought; patience and a willingness to experiment may open up whole new vistas of sexual pleasure. Many chemotherapy patients turn to self-stimulation and find it a reasonable solution to needs that might otherwise go completely unfulfilled at this time.

Starting up new relationships is difficult for anyone but can pose a special challenge for people on chemotherapy. You may feel reluctant and awkward about bringing up the subject of your cancer and its therapy at first. But once the discussion has begun, communicating your feelings can help strip away superficialities and cultivate a closeness that might not otherwise have occurred or taken forever to develop. Cancer patients have the ultimate satisfaction of knowing that they are loved for themselves, not just for the way they look or for their ability to become parents.

OUTSIDE HELP

Sometimes the chemo-related sexual changes are such that they can't be dealt with between partners. At times, referral to a sex clinic or therapist may be in order. But often just talking things over with a sympathetic person can be a help. A nurse, a social worker, other patients, support groups, or your gynecologist or urologist will help you find some answers. A sensitive oncologist may be able to answer your needs for sex counseling or information; he or she may also be able to suggest material for home reading. However, many patients find it difficult to bring up the subject with their oncologists, who rarely bring it up themselves.

Lari Wenzel, former director of the Cancer Information Service at the Comprehensive Cancer Center for the state of Florida, says:

> "I think the problem is much greater than people will admit. The problem starts when the physician doesn't ask, and most patients aren't going to bring it up. It's not a routine part of your physical exam. And unless you have a very close relationship with the doctor and you are very assertive, it's just a problem that's not acknowledged the way it should be."

Both patient and doctor may feel awkward and uncomfortable discussing intimate sexual details. Physicians often are not equipped or eager to do sex counseling, or they don't realize that sexuality can be a concern at this time. Dr. William Grace, an oncologist at St. Vincent's Hospital in New York, says: "A lot of people just resign themselves and say, 'Well, I'm not going to be sexually active at this time.' A lot of people don't want to talk about it; it's very hush-hush. I'd say only about 10 percent of my patients bring it up, and when they do, it's usually with a nurse, who then tells me."

Fortunately, many problems have simple solutions. "A lot of patients' sexual problems are related to the side effects of chemotherapy," continues Dr. Grace; here the oncologist's medical skills can surely help. "They may have painful intercourse due to vaginal dryness or stomatitis. If there is an infection presents—infections like trichomona and candida have an increased risk at this time—we treat that." If there is fatigue, nausea, constipation, or diarrhea, you can take medications and measures that reduce them too.

STERILITY AND MENOPAUSE

For many chemotherapy patients, the drugs' impact on their reproductive system is a discrete, though important, issue closely related to their ability to express themselves sexually and to their feelings about themselves as complete human beings. Some chemotherapy drugs—primarily the alkylating agents such as chlorambucil and Cytoxan—are well known for their ability to reduce sperm counts or sperm vitality in men. These drugs plus two others—busulfan and vinblastine—are also known to suppress ovarian function and menstruation in women.

As a result, the chemotherapy patient runs the risk of becoming infertile or subfertile during therapy. This condition may be temporary and disappear after treatment is over. But it can take a long time to reverse itself, and it sometimes never does, or does so incompletely.

It is probably that the total amount of these drugs and length of time you take them play key roles in the incidence and reversibility of early menopause and fertility problems. Permanent sterility is most common in patients who receive high-dose long-term chemotherapy, such as for Hodgkin's disease, and less common in low-dose short-term chemo plans such as adjuvant treatment for breast cancer.

Sterility is more of a long-term problem that an immediate one because conception is inadvisable during chemotherapy. This is primarily because anticancer drugs have the potential to cause birth defects (*teratogenesis*) and mutations in offspring that are exposed to the drugs while in the womb, and as sperm or eggs even before conception. However, there is no firm proof that the danger occurs with every drug and so, as Drs. Holland and Frei point out in *Cancer Medicine*, this problem is hard to assess. There are patients who while on chemotherapy have produced apparently healthy offspring, but some warn that even in seemingly healthy babies chromosomal damage may be latent and not show up until some future generation. Most of the danger appears to be in the first trimester of pregnancy, and the overall risk in later trimesters appears the same as under normal conditions. Nevertheless, many physicians feel the risk is high enough to recommend that their patients use contraception during chemotherapy. Dr. Grace says, "Chemotherapy is not a form of birth control. It is difficult to get pregnant while on chemo, but not impossible."

If a woman is pregnant at the time of diagnosis, she is usually not given chemotherapy unless her life is in immediate danger from the disease, and chemotherapy has a chance to produce a cure or remission. Breast feeding may be hazardous to the baby if the mother is on chemo. Sometimes an abortion is advised if a pregnancy is already established but, again, the decision is not clear-cut. Patients should discuss the possible risks with their doctors. Women patients who are sexually active and who miss a period should have a pregnancy test as soon as possible.

In the past, there was a special concern when the patient had cancer of a reproductive organ such as the breast, which is sensitive to the levels of hormones in the body. Since pregnancy changes these levels, it was theorized that a pregnancy could stimulate the growth of cancer and precipitate a recurrence. However, recent studies show that pregnancy does not significantly raise the rate of recurrence.

Sterility, or the possibility of it, is more of an issue for some patients and their spouses than for others. Age, former plans, and the presence of previous children affect its importance:

"I don't like it at all. My wife's reaction isn't good either.
The old affection isn't there now that we can't have
children together. Sure we have sex, but it isn't like it
used to be. The little things—like stroking—are left out.
My wife is going to a psychiatrist. I go out a few nights
a week—not for a one-night stand, but to get attention
and affection and to boost my ego a little. I'm a very
sensual, romantic guy at heart and that part of me is not
being expressed while my wife isn't interested."

The possibility of being sterile is not a major problem for
me, since I have no overwhelming desire to have children. But
it does seem odd—extending your own life in exchange for a
potential child. At the moment it doesn't bother me—except
that I do like to have options, whether I intend to exercise them
or not, and this may have removed one of them. Now that
having my own child may be out of the question, I sometimes
feel a pang of regret. But who knows? I may be as fertile as
I ever was, and it may never even be an issue.

If you are still of child-bearing age, you should talk over
family planning and contraception with your physician, nurse,
or social worker. (The pill and IUD are usually not recommended for chemotherapy patients.) This should be done *before*
you begin chemotherapy. Although sterility or subfertility may
be reversible, it may not be. Therefore, male chemotherapy
patients are often advised to visit a sperm bank while they still
have viable sperm. Should the chemotherapy leave them permanently sterile, they may still be able to father children via
artificial insemination. Women about to undergo chemotherapy
unfortunately do not have an equivalent option at this time and
are usually counseled about the possiblity of adoption. Still,
these alternatives leave much to be desired, especially for young
single adults who want children, and for couples whose families
are not yet complete. Anxiety and regret over this loss can spill
into many aspects of their lives and sometimes professional
counseling helps people adapt.

For men, cytotoxic agents kill the rapidly producing sperm.
This reduction in the production of sperm is not of itself directly
responsible for reducing either the desire or the ability to have
sex from a physiological point of view. Theoretically, unless
"feminizing" hormone therapy is also begin given, a man's
testosterone levels are not affected and he can still achieve and

maintain an erection and ejaculation. An infertile man can still enjoy sex, and so can his partner. However, no one is sure about this, and in reality, some men do find that their libidos are lessened during chemotherapy. (It is uncertain whether this is due to physical or emotional factors.)

It's quite different for a woman, whose reproductive system, with its delicately balanced menstrual cycle, is much more complex than a man's. A woman is born with her total supply of ova, or eggs; unlike a man's sperm, they are not manufactured constantly in the body—they mature, one at a time per cycle, during ovulation. A woman on chemo undergoes estrogen withdrawal and possibly other hormonal changes. These changes prevent the egg from maturing and cause menstrual irregularities, and women can undergo real, verifiable physical and emotional changes. Aside from the discomfort and embarrassment of hot flashes, women experience profuse sweating, vaginal infections, dry or sore vaginas, uncomfortable intercourse, dizziness, difficulty in breathing, mood swings, and a more than usual uncertainty about the possibility of pregnancy. If hormonal therapy is administered simultaneously or sequentially to chemotherapy, these problems are compounded, and women may experience signs of masculinization such as excess facial and bodily hair, and a lowered voice.

These effects may be almost immediate or take several months to become evident; other changes in the vagina, cervix, skin, and bones can occur eventually if the menopause becomes permanent. All of these sex and hormone-related side effects can reduce the quality of sex and the quality of life for women during and after chemotherapy. Even if their periods do not stop completely, some women miss the rhythm of a physical phenomenon that has occurred so regularly up to then.

Women may be thrust into artificial menopause, often at a very young age. Doctors don't often warn women about this eventuality and often fail to realize, or believe, or accept the amount of distress this can cause. Here are two women's experiences:

"I had lost my period completely about six months after beginning the chemo; it got irregular, and very light, and then stopped. I'm on tamoxifen now, which suppresses the hormone production in the body. When I get a hot flash, my body temperature goes skyhigh and my face gets beet red. Sometimes my emotions will set it off. The sweat pours down, and I feel like I can't breathe— like I'm having an anxiety attack. Then there's the erratic behavior . . . I hope this is temporary, as my doctor says. I'm a young woman, yet."

"When I went into chemical menopause, my doctor told me it was my imagination. Right! There in the middle of winter I was sitting in church, fanning myself like crazy, turning bright red. My periods never came back, even though my doctor said there was enough estrogen so they might. I have no symptoms now; I'm not uncomfortable with it."

Health professionals, in their powerlessness to treat menopause effectively and safely, sometimes dismiss its symptoms as "psychosomatic" or tell patients to grin and bear it. Estrogen has been widely used in the past to relieve the symptoms of menopause. But estrogen replacement therapy has been linked with several forms of cancer and other diseases, and so some say is not advisable for any woman, but especially not for a cancer patient. There are other ways that you can deal with the physical and emotional changes brought about by this side effect. You can contact women's support groups whose members have gone through menopause themselves. You can refer to the books on this subject listed in the Sources Section. One of them, *Coping with a Hysterectomy* by Susanne Morgan, explains how to make "home-brew estrogen." This involves a general change in life habits that encourage overall health and the body's own production of estrogen. The plan includes exercise, stress reduction, nutrition, and diet. Experience has shown, for instance, that symptoms are reduced when women cut down on sugar, coffee, and salt consumption, and take supplements such as calcium, and vitamins B, E, and C. Ms. Morgan also discusses the importance of remaining sexually active—it is a common misconception that sexual desire diminishes after menopause. But this may be in part a self-fulfilling prophecy (use it or lose it).

CHAPTER 14

Other Side Effects

BLADDER AND KIDNEY PROBLEMS

Cyclophosphamide (Cytoxan) can cause acute, noninfectious (hemorrhagic) cystitis. Since 70 percent of this drug is excreted by the kidneys, the bladder is given plenty of exposure to this drug, and it is thought that the cystitis results from the drug acting directly on the mucosa that lines the bladder. Chronic bladder irritation can cause scar tissue to form and as a result the bladder is able to hold less and there is the need for more frequent urination. In this rare complication of therapy, the symptoms are painful, frequent urination, urgency of urination, and blood in the urine.

Cystitis seems to appear to be more of a danger in those who receive large doses of this drug intravenously, who are on prolonged therapy, or who do not drink enough fluids. It is recommended therefore that anyone who is receiving this drug should drink as much liquid as possible—up to three quarts a day, which may be in the form of water or other beverages such as soda, juices, or Popsicles or Jell-O.

The onset of the symptoms may occur as early as twenty-four hours after the first drug dose or be delayed until several weeks after the end of the treatment. Acute symptoms usually go away when the drug is stopped, but slight bleeding may persist for months. Treatment for noninfectious cystitis that is not severe consists of medication; when it is more serious, surgery may be be necessary. The same symptoms of noninfectious cystitis may indicate infectious cystitis, which may be treated with antibiotics.

Other drugs given to treat cancer can act on the kidneys (renal toxicity). These include cisplatin, dacarbazine, daunorubicin, doxorubicin, lomustine, Methotrexate, mitocycin, and Mithramycin. Kidney damage can be serious and sometimes is severe and leads to fatal kidney failure. However, it may be reversible if caught early enough. As is beneficial against bladder toxicity, drinking large quantities of liquids can prevent these problems from occurring or at least minimize them. In some cases and with some drugs, large doses of vitamin C, mannitol, or sodium bicarbonate have been used in an attempt to further minimize the risks. (Doxorubicin in the system creates red-colored urine, which lasts only one or two days and is not serious.) Renal function may also be affected by the remnants of dead cancer cells themselves that pass through the kidneys. Drinking plenty of liquids usually forestalls any problems, but allopurinol may also be prescribed to prevent problems in patients with leukemia and lymphomas, where large numbers of cancer cells are destroyed.

FLULIKE SYMPTOMS

While on chemotherapy, patients sometimes feel like they have the flu—an all-over achiness in their muscles and/or bones, possibly a fever and chills, or a feeling of general malaise. They may indeed have caught an infectious virus, since their immune systems are likely to be compromised. However, some drugs used in chemotherapy can themselves cause these symptoms to appear when no infection is actually present. Any of the antibiotics can give you flulike symptoms, as can cytarabine, dacarbazine, Thiotepa, and VP-16. Vincristine and vinblastine can give you an all-over achy feeling. These symptoms are temporary and pass within days of treatment. They should respond to the usual nostrums prescribed for the flu: Tylenol, fluids, rest.

HEART PROBLEMS

Heart damage (cardiotoxicity) is the principal dose-limiting side effect of two antibiotics: Daunorubicin and doxorubicin (Adriamycin). Prednisone may also damage the heart. When cardiotoxicity occurs, the drugs' effects are usually cumulative; they can lead to chronic congestive heart failure which may be progressive and eventually fatal. The onset of the symptoms may not occur until long after the drug has been begun— usually two weeks to six months after therapy has been completed. Cumulative congestive heart failure may be irreversible, but it may respond to drug therapy with digitalis and diuretics.

In the rarer acute form of cardiotoxicity, the effects on the heart occur during or shortly after the drug is administered. The effects usually reverse quickly without serious complications and are usually not considered a reason to stop the drug. At one time 75 percent of those who experienced cardiotoxicity died, but it is being recognized earlier and treated more successfully. Studies are underway to improve early diagnosis even more and perhaps prevent cardiotoxicity's occurrence through blocking chemicals. Vitamin E, for example, has been found to protect the heart from Adriamycin in animals and may prove to do the same in humans. There is an investigational drug that might replace Adriamycin in effectiveness and has less toxicity. For now the only preventive measures are for the oncologist to give the drugs very slowly and for the patient to have a good, strong heart to begin with.

LIVER PROBLEMS

Many of the drugs used in cancer chemotherapy produce some degree of liver impairment (hepatotoxicity); most are difficult to measure and unnoticeable because of the liver's ability to withstand a tremendous amount of abuse. And abuse is what it gets during chemotherapy because the liver works overtime to detoxify harmful substances before they are excreted from the body.

Methotrexate and mercaptopurine are the two drugs usually

associated with cirrhosis and fibrosis (scarring) of the liver, especially during long-term use. Other drugs such as asparaginase, carmustine, Cytoxan, dacarbazine, doxorubicin (Adriamycin), mithramycin, steptozocin, and thioguanine have also been implicated in liver dysfunction. Combination chemotherapy, preexisting liver dysfunction, and alcohol intake can compound these drugs' effects on the liver, which may become evident within one or two months after treatment, or as late as two years afterward.

LUNG PROBLEMS

Lung damage (pulmonary toxicity) is a rare side effect, although many drugs have the potential to cause it. Busulfan, carmustine, chlorambucil, Cytoxan, bleomycin, and Methotrexate have been known to cause lung damage in a small percentage of patients. The damage, which is a kind of scarring (fibrosis), is characterized by a dry cough, shortness of breath, high pulse, and a low grade fever. Pulmonary damage may be reversible with time when the drug is stopped early and corticosteroids are administered. However, there is irreversible damage in some people and as a result, they are chronically short of breath and must change their life-styles accordingly.

Pulmonary toxicity may occur after the first treatment; this is usually due to a hypersensitivity to the drug and is helped by corticosteroids. However, it may not become evident until long after chemotherapy, even years after the therapy has ended.

Because this reaction is so rare and the early symptoms subtle or unreported, lung damage may be undetected until quite late. Dr. William Grace, an oncologist at St. Vincent's Hospital in New York, says:

> "Early diagnosis is the key. If it goes too far there may be no coming back. If a patient has symptoms and an X ray shows nothing, you go on to test for pulmonary functions. I think that what you often see is a busy oncologist who keeps giving the drug because toxicity is not detected soon enough. Subclinical or early forms of toxicity are often not recognized."

NERVOUS SYSTEM PROBLEMS

There are several chemotherapy drugs that are known for their effects on the nervous system.

As a result of taking vincristine or vinblastine, patients may experience nerve damage in the hands and feet, the symptoms of which are a tingling or a numbness in the fingertips and/or toes. There may be damage to the nerves that control the action of the intestines, which results in constipation, sluggish bowels, or a coliclike pain. Sometimes the facial nerve is affected, and there is a deep aching pain in the jaw or in the throat. A loss of deep tendon reflexes or increased motor weakness causes foot or wrist drop, difficulty walking or rising from a chair, clumsiness, or a loss of coordination. In addition, the impotence of which some men complain is possibly a result of nerve damage.

Vincristine was part of my chemo protocol, and I did experience some tingling and numbness in my fingers and toes. It came on so gradually I barely noticed it. It was winter, so I thought maybe the cold had something to do with it. I never would have said anything if my oncologist hadn't eventually asked me about it. I got quite constipated for a while, but we don't know whether that was from the drugs or from my different diet and decrease in exercise. I noticed one foot would sort of lag behind when I walked, but I thought I was just tired.

In addition to these fairly concrete, measurable signs of neurotoxicity, there is a whole constellation of others which are vague and much harder to put a finger on. They can result in a mental muzziness or cloudiness, a feeling of being doped up, off balance, and not "with it." Some people on chemo, myself included, just feel slower, duller, and clumsier mentally and physically. Though it is difficult to distinguish the emotional and physical contributors from the direct pharmacological culprits, certain drugs are associated with these effects.

Vincristine and vinblastine, for example, can cause muscle weakness; vincristine in addition can cause muscle cramps. Both drugs have been known to cause mental depression. Asparaginase may affect the nervous system by causing mental depression, hallucinations, confusion, lethargy, and nervousness. Procarbazine's effects include depression, tiredness, agitation, dizziness, hallucinations, confusion, weakness, and unsteadiness. Floxuridine can cause depression and lethargy; mitotane, depression, drowsiness, and tremors; Thiotepa, dizziness; 5-fluorouracil can also cause clumsiness and a little bit of slowness. Dr. Grace says, "Since neurological damage is not a well-known effect, it is often not recognized or looked for. Some people say they become complete klutzes—they just fall down. People also can't do serial sevens—subtracting seven from one hundred, then seven from that result, then seven from that, and so on. They can't balance their checkbooks, or themselves." Three patients relate their neurological side effects:

> "I lost my balance a few times, and I actually fell. My legs got so wobbly, like butter. My doctor called it 'sea legs'—he said that many patients get it. It's been nearly two years since my last treatment, and I still feel like my legs haven't gotten their strength back. I still feel like they could buckle under me any time. I'm a forty-four-year-old person! Sometimes I walk like an old person—with little tiny steps. My doctor says they should get stronger; he's heard of this."

> "While on chemo, I lost my equilibrium. I tripped and broke my leg two months after chemo began; that healed well. Several months after that I lost my balance, and broke my shoulder and arm. And then I fell in my kitchen—I fractured my ribs and tore a muscle in my arm. Then I punctured my eardrum with a Q-Tip because I again lost my balance and felt uncoordinated. I lost my hearing in that ear. People said they used to cry when they saw me."

> "I used to flounder for words, have trouble finishing sentences. I also found I was forgetting things—I'm not talking about forgetting keys—I would forget entire conversations."

With cisplatin another side effect on the nervous system occurs. This takes the form of ototoxicity, where there is a hearing loss, and/or tinnitus (ringing in the ears). When there is a loss of hearing, it's usually only in the high frequencies. Ototoxicity occurs in approximately 30 percent of the patients who receive cisplatin. It may also occur in patients receiving mechlorethamine. A testicular cancer patient says:

"I had a dramatic hearing loss for a while, which worried me because so much of my job entails telephone contact. I've gotten some hearing back, but telephone conversations are still very difficult. The doctors aren't sure whether it will ever come back, and they say if not maybe a hearing aid will help later on."

"I sit at my desk in the dead of winter, in a high-rise building in the middle of the city; there is construction going on outside, and I could swear there's a nest full of blue jays fighting right outside my window. Every once in a while in the evening I'll be sitting listening to records or reading the paper and I'll turn to my wife, just to be sure about this, and ask her, 'There is not a nest of birds fighting outside the window, is there?' She'll say, 'No—it's back again isn't it?'"

Stool softeners, laxatives, enemas, and an increase in dietary fiber are used to counteract sluggish bowels caused by neurotoxicity. The risk of ototoxicity from cisplatin may be minimized by using forced diuresis—massive doses of fluid given intravenously before and after the drug—and if the drug is given very slowly. Hearing tests can be administered regularly to prevent severe, irreversible hearing loss. Exercise may reduce the risk of other forms of neurotoxicity because when you exercise you're using the nervous system. "I don't know of any hard data," says Dr. Grace, "but I will tell you this: I see less neurotoxicity in active people. Those who are most inactive have more problems with clumsiness and confusion. Practice makes perfect—you get more coordinated by being physically active. I do tell them, though, to avoid sports that require skills or are dangerous, I recommend vigorous walking, for instance, and advise them to stay off bikes and be careful when walking down stairs." Other than that, he says, "There is not much you can do for neurotoxicity, other than reduce the drugs. The doctor has to be very careful in addressing this toxicity."

Neurotoxicity is for the most part temporary and reversible. (Those who undergo therapy with vincristine or vinblastine in high doses or over a long period of time are at a higher risk to develop neurotoxicity that is less reversible.) Its symptoms may peak a few days after a treatment and then gradually subside. They usually disappear completely after treatment has been concluded. But this may take up to two years and in some patients they may never go away completely.

Neurotoxicity can be dangerous. Patients should tell their doctors if any of the above symptoms occur. Though tingling toes may seem like "nothing," they could indicate more serious nerve damage that should be caught early.

SLEEP DISTURBANCES

Nighttime is often a difficult time for the chemo patient, and for many reasons. Some drugs are directly blamed for causing nervousness or agitation. The corticosteroids such as prednisone are notorious for their stimulating effects which may be advantageous during the day, but disastrous at night. Many people have trouble falling asleep while taking these drugs, but they are unaware that there may be pharmacological reasons and blame their sleeplessness on everything else. Another drug, procarbazine, is known to cause insomnia and nightmares.

Pain and discomfort seem to grow and fears and problems loom larger in the still of the night, when daytime activities are not around to distract you. Surgical pain, emotional stress, and sleeplessness can feed upon each other in a vicious cycle. It may be even more difficult to sleep if you are being treated in the hospital and sleeping in a strange bed, with nurses and staff buzzing around, your roommate groaning or snoring, and machines whirring or clanking.

Any sleeping problems should be discussed with your nurse or doctor, so he or she can begin to help you do something about them. If you are taking a corticosteroid like prednisone, your oncologist might suggest that you take the drug early in the day in order to give the stimulating effects time to wear off before bedtime. Taking measures to relieve any emotional anxieties that are coming between you and a good night's sleep is another good initial step. Establishing a ritual usually helps lull people to sleep. Reading, listening to soft music, watching TV, taking a hot bath or shower, having a soothing massage, doing some deep breathing, or stretching or relaxation exercises—even the proverbial glass of warm milk are several

conservative, nondrug methods you can use to help you get to
sleep. You may have not needed them in the past but that's no
reason not to explore them now, and to use them for as long
as you need them. Nor should you hesitate to ask for or use
some kind of sleeping pill to get you through a particularly
tough time. Sometimes a single good night's sleep can make
all the difference in your outlook and general well-being. Sleep
is especially important for the chemo patient because it enables
you to better face the next day's challenges.

CHAPTER 15

Emotional Impact

As a cancer chemotherapy patient, your emotional balance receives a terrific one-two punch: one, the diagnosis of a disease that is highly symbolic and threatens your very life; two, a long-lasting toxic treatment that threatens the quality of your life but whose effectiveness is uncertain. Cancer patients face both their own reactions and those of others to their disease and its treatment. They are called upon to adjust to new environments and new people; they must find ways of dealing with big and little stresses and responsibilities. It is no surprise that for many patients the emotional stress of the disease and its treatment is far more devastating than the physical stress.

Just as no two patients will have the exact same physical response to chemotherapy, so are people's emotional reactions and resulting behavior as individual as fingerprints. Unlike the physical side effects, which are concrete, measurable, and observable by others, the emotional consequences of cancer and chemotherapy are not tangible, easily measurable, seen, or felt by anyone else. This does not mean, however, that they are not real or that they have to be endured.

The emotional reactions of cancer patients vary:

"I can't really describe how I felt. I think I just didn't want to believe it. I just felt so deserted that day."

"I had adjusted pretty well to the mastectomy—I was glad I still had my eyes, my arms, my legs—you know, I didn't really miss having a breast, and the rehabilitation wouldn't be too involved. But the chemo really blew my mind. I had a fatalistic attitude at first."

"I was an ultramarathon runner and found myself barely able to do a ten-minute mile. When my doctor told me the final diagnosis, I had an out-of-body experience. I felt like I was viewing the situation as if it were someone else being told. After about ten minutes I came back to earth and started talking to people about my options. Soon after that I started poring through the medical literature. I went straight to the acceptance stage; I became galvanized into action."

"A lot of people look at you and say, 'God, I'm so sorry.' And deep down inside they're thinking, 'Thank God it isn't me.' I would too—I'll be honest about it. If there were some way I could have given it to someone else, I would have."

MAKING SENSE OF IT ALL

Dr. Judith Bukberg, chief of Consultation-Liaison Psychiatry at New York's St. Vincent's Hospital, who specializes in treating cancer patients, says:

"I think there's too much stoicism in the world. People seem to have the idea that because this is real—because something real and bad is happening to them—that all kinds of emotional reactions are to be tolerated. That's ridiculous. Sure, you have a reason to be depressed, but that doesn't mean you can't do something about it.

"People also don't want to upset other people—either their families, friends, or doctors—and so they put on a great face to the world, and meanwhile God knows what's going on inside of them. People want to protect each other, but it isn't always helpful in the long run—either to themselves or their relationships."

That cancer patients do suffer a lot of stress and emotional turmoil was shown in a study done by the Psychosocial Collaborative Oncology Group. The investigators found that 47 percent of the patients who were interviewed and tested showed serious emotional turmoil, mostly depression or anxiety, in trying to adjust to their illness.

The emotional impact of cancer and its treatment—how it influences your behavior, work, social interaction, and overall quality of life—are called "psychosocial effects." The study of the psychosocial impact of cancer and chemotherapy is still in its infancy. Its importance has only recently been recognized. Nevertheless, some basic patterns have emerged as to what emotions patients are likely to feel, when they are most likely to feel them, and what can be done to help patients cope with their emotions. By becoming familiar with the way others have seen things, you may develop a framework that makes some sense out of your own experience. By becoming acquainted with various probabilities and possibilities you can begin to get a handle on your emotions and thus are in a better position to cope yourself. You will be aware of the availability of others who can help.

Once concept of the impact of cancer and chemotherapy involves thinking in terms of the emotional stages that many people go through when faced with death or any stressful, unpleasant situation. You will probably recognize this pattern in yourself or in your family.

· *Denial*. No not me! It's all a mistake. I don't believe it; this can't be happening. I don't want to think about it.

· *Anger*. Why me? What did I do to deserve this? Why not somebody else?

· *Bargaining or Guilt*. I promise I'll do anything to be cured—I'll change my life, my personality, I'll be "good."

· *Depression*. I feel so low and discouraged. Nothing matters, nothing will help, what's the use?

· *Acceptance*. Okay, this is the way it is. Now let's get the show on the road and do something about it.

The five-stage cycle begins around the time of diagnosis; it continues into the therapy and persists long thereafter. With each subsequent stressful event such as surgery, the beginning of chemotherapy, or the failure of chemotherapy, the cycle is repeated. Some people may need to skip stages, or to remain in one stage longer than others. Denial, for instance, (which can masquerade as healthy optimism and vice versa), was once thought best gotten over quickly. Now mental health experts think it may be an appropriate, helpful stage that should not be rushed. Richard S. Lazarus writes in Paul Ahmed's book *Living and Dying with Cancer* that denial or self-deception is "often a valuable initial form of coping, occurring at a time when the person is confused and weakened and therefore unable to act constructively and realistically." Denial is a way to buy time, to recoup from the shock so we can digest the news and gradually come to deal with the threat. When our reasoning powers return, we will be able to act rationally. Some people just need more time.

In the hospital after my surgery, people were amazed at my good spirits. An army of friends practically never went home, and the jokes were flying fast and furiously. "The Perle Mesta of the cancer ward" is what they called me, but I realize now it was good old denial doing its job and helping me survive.

Living with surgical scars, pain, and loss of functioning, going for chemotherapy treatments and suffering the side effects—all can be more distressing because they remind us of our situation and so make denial harder. Every time I went to the oncologist for treatment, I was reminded that I had cancer. It wasn't only the side effects I knew the drugs would bring that made me not want to go. It was that gut-wrenching kick to my psyche ... I'm going here because I have cancer and may die.

Another approach to making sense out of emotional turmoil centers on the four general issues of alienation, mutilation, mortality, and vulnerability. As is explained in *Coping with Cancer*, a handbook published by the National Cancer Institute geared toward health care professionals, most cancer patients at some point are confronted by these basic issues, from which spring a host of emotional reactions.

Alienation. Patients who feel alienated have fears of abandonment, unacceptability, and isolation—they feel alone in the world, unconnected, apart, and unable to relate to other human beings. Patients' feelings may originate within themselves or be based upon real situations and the very real reactions of others. Cancer is a disease with many negative connotations.

Many of these are unfounded or exaggerated, but this does not diminish their impact. Chemo patients may feel sorry for themselves and shut out the rest of the world. They may think their diagnosis is a punishment for past wrongdoings or personality traits, or an automatic death sentence, and they may break off contact from loved ones as a preparation for the final separation. (A chemotherapy patient may indeed be *physically* alone and apart because of time spent in hospitals or undergoing treatment, or being away from work or being sick and unable to socialize.) People may withdraw emotionally from chemotherapy patients for various reasons, including fear that the patient may die, feelings of guilt, anger, and resentment, and fear that the disease is contagious.

Patients and others may fall prey to the nonsensical myths and superstitions that surround cancer—that it is something of which to be ashamed, that it is a form of punishment for being "a bad person," that it is contagious. They may be embarrassed by a change in bodily functions and reluctant to expose them to others. For example:

> "We call it 'the big C.' Amazing how you put cute little nicknames on everything. Cancer is a very difficult word to say. And when you tell people you have it they can't look you in the face."

> "While I was on chemo, I would not permit anyone to kiss me, or to come too close to me. I just felt—and they also helped me feel—like a leper. I would never permit anyone to eat from my food, even my husband. Except when we went out to a restaurant once a week with other people, he would offer me food, and I would take it from his fork. I would subject him to something that I thought was contagious because I wanted them to see that he was not afraid."

Mutilation. Many aspects of cancer and its treatments are disfiguring and invasive; patients may feel mutilated as a result of surgery, for example, and mourn the loss of parts of their bodies, their attractiveness, and their abilities to function. They may not feel "whole" and suffer from changes in body image. And chemotherapy does change body images, when large amounts of weight are lost and gained, and when hair is lost, or when people feel they just don't look like themselves. These changes are even more devastating when they are visible to others, and when treatment of cancer of the reproductive organs leave patients feeling that they are less than a woman or not quite a man. I, for example, would avoid looking in the mirror, although there was a strange attraction to do it, a fascination— like rubbernecking at an accident. I couldn't believe the scar, the bald head, the lack of eyelashes and eyebrows, the circles under the eyes, the pallor. I'd feel where my breast had been— gone. Touch where my hair had been—gone. Who was this person? I felt like such a phoney. I had to wear a wig and a prosthesis just to be "normal," to be accepted.

Mortality. Cancer patients become more aware of the inevitability of death—their own, whether from their cancer or another cause. Death is no longer the abstract philosophical concept it is for most other people—it is a reality. Mortality is an unavoidable issue regardless of the prognosis and goal of the therapy—be it cure, remission, or palliation.

Most days I'd chug along just fine, even though it was in the back of my mind. But every once in a while it would get to me: *This disease could kill me.* I'd flip out and scream and cry from fear and remorse. I'd imagine my own death and rage against the unfairness of it all. I wonder what the neighbors thought. I didn't want to die!

Vulnerability. Many cancer patients become distressed by the loss of control over their lives and their health. They hate feeling dependent, helpless—at the mercy of their disease and other people. They feel a loss of self-esteem and self-confidence, which is worsened by the fatigue, debility, weakness, and consequent inability to perform their usual functions. Feelings of worthlessness may surface. The uncertainty of treatment, the duration of the disease, and the steady stream of side effects create an atmosphere of unending sickness. For some people the fact that the cancer itself is defined as a disease of uncontrolled growth reinforces feelings of the loss of control.

"Every time another side effect appeared, it was another blow. I kept feeling worse and worse; I worried what could go wrong next and where it would all end."

"I'm not afraid of pain, or of death. I'm afraid of being disabled . . . of being stuck in bed, not even able to wash myself."

Every patient will not necessarily go through the full spectrum of possible emotions; nor will he or she feel them all at once. At various times some feelings will recede and others will come into the foreground. Studies of cancer patients have found that people (except for those with lung cancer) are usually most vulnerable psychologically three to four months after diagnosis. As a result of her experience in social work, Grace Christ finds it useful to think in terms of a series of potential crisis points. Chemotherapy patients and their families are under the most stress during these times and must perform adaptive tasks at each of them if and when they occur: (1) the time of diagnosis, (2) the beginning of treatment, (3) negative physical reactions to treatment (side effects), (4) failure of conventional treatment, (5) the end of a treatment protocol, (6) the recurrence or metastasis of the disease, (7) the beginning of investigational treatment, (8) the end of active treatment, and (9) terminal illness.

HOW YOU COPE

Chances are if you cope well generally you will manage to cope with chemo too. People who cope best tend to be flexible and have the ability to shift their perspectives and see situations in new ways that allow problems to be solved. Other useful characteristics include independence, but a willingness to lean on others when necessary; cooperativeness without complete passivity; and a positive attitude. People who cope poorly are often already in emotional turmoil from personal problems and disrupted family background, have a pessimistic attitude, expect no help from others, have poor self-esteem, and rely on tension-reducing devices rather than activity to change the source of tension.

Dr. Bukberg points out that what is especially stressful for one person may be less so for another, and that how—and how well—you cope with cancer and chemotherapy depends upon three basic factors: how much stress you are actually under; how you perceive the stress; and your own unique coping style, abilities, and support system. Age, sex, personality, intelligence, values and beliefs, the type and extent of the cancer and treatment, what they mean to you, and the quality of your relationships with others will enter into the coping process.

HOW MUCH STRESS?

Some therapies themselves are indeed more stressful than others. There may be more toxic effects and more physical and thus more emotional stress. A patient's life may be quite disrupted due to physical symptoms or the location and timing of the treatment. Some cancers are more malignant than others, and some prognoses are worse. There may be other stresses outside of the treatment, or due to the treatment (such as financial problems or family troubles) that are already straining the patient's coping abilities.

HOW DO YOU PERCEIVE STRESS?

A situation such as chemotherapy treatment may be perceived as a threat, a source of pain, a challenge, or as an attempt to help. Some people are much more able to contain anxiety, or they just don't get anxious easily. Others become fearful and nervous very readily. Also, your past medical history can influence the way you feel about medical treatment; if you've already had a bad experience with a certain procedure, you will be more anxious about it than someone who hasn't. "People who come from loving trusting families," says Dr. Bukberg, "have more trust in health professionals and are more able to put their lives in their hands."

HOW DO YOU HANDLE STRESS?

Dr. Bukberg defines coping as "something that an individual does—either as an automatic response or as a thought-out, planned response to a stress—that is designed to decrease the amount of emotional upheaval, and/or in some way to affect the environment to reduce the stress." Each person has certain coping mechanisms—a certain way to deal with things—as a part of his or her personality. People have tendencies to respond one way or another, based upon what else has happened to them in the past and what has worked under previous conditions. Broadly speaking, people cope actively or passively. As Dr. Bukberg observes, referring to a concept introduced by Dr. Lipowski, some people tend to avoid all kinds of stress—they deny or minimize a problem. They may disregard the facts, the true meaning of a piece of information, or their emotional state. At the other end of the spectrum, some people become "hypervigilant." They are anxiety-prone, intellectualizing, and somewhat obsessive—they loathe ambiguity and uncertainty, and they want to know as much as they can and become totally involved in their treatment.

Some people rely on their religious convictions. Others become stoical or rationalize their cancer by saying there are people who are worse off. Some merely defer thinking about it until they are strong enough to cope. Some, accepting every blow, attempt to treat their problems lightly and try to shrug everything off with jokes. Others are problem solvers. There are many, many ways of coping, and usually a person will need to combine several of the ways to get the best effect.

All these mechanisms do help us relieve stress. But they may not work as well as they have for different circumstances in the past. They may work temporarily, or partially, but not enough to reduce our fears, anxieties, or depression to a bearable level. If your usual ways of coping are not working now, or not working as well as you'd like them to, perhaps this is the time to expand your coping repertoire.

For any given stressful situation, there are usually several options, some or all of which you may not be aware. Here, for example, is a stressful situation experienced by many chemo patients: You are not happy with your oncologist—he is abrupt and cool, he doesn't treat you like a human being or ever tell you anything. This is making you anxious, and you are tired of feeling like a pincushion with a checkbook instead of a patient. Your usual passive, accepting, or minimizing attitude is no longer working—What do you do? Dr. Bukberg says:

> "There are three options. You can do something behaviorally such as talking to your doctor about it or changing to another doctor. Or you could do something cognitive, which would be to try to understand for example, that he may be upset at having to cause discomfort to people, or at having so many people to see that he can't get more involved—in some way redefine the situation so it is more manageable to you. Or you could do something that is directly tension reducing such as relaxation techniques or hypnosis, where you are primarily reducing the tension that is aroused by the situation."

No coping mechanism is intrinsically "good" or "bad," "right" or "wrong." A mechanism may, however, not be *useful* in a particular situation. When your usual style of coping is not working well enough—when it does not solve a problem, or at least bring stress down to a tolerable level—it is time for a change. Change doesn't mean admitting that you were "wrong." Your favorite sneakers may serve you well in weather when you can wear them; they may be comfortable and familiar. But comes a snowstorm and they do not work well. Learning how to cope better may take practice. It may take work. It may be painful and slow in spite of your immediate need for it: Trading in your old ways of thinking and acting for new patterns is not easy. But coping can be learned just like any other skill.

In addition, the changes that chemotherapy puts you through may not seem pleasant at the time, but many people find it is ultimately a positive experience and feel it changes them for the better. Patients say it can be a tremendous personal growth experience. Dealing with their troubles in a time of crisis makes them more mature, more tolerant, more understanding of others, and feeling more—not less—in command of their lives. Their relationships with others can improve, too, as loved ones grow along with and become closer to the patient.

IMPROVING YOUR COPING SKILLS

There are four basic, interrelated areas for you to explore if you want to expand your coping repertoire—attitude, communication, education, and support services. Chapters 5 through 9 will also give you some ideas for supporting your mind, body, and spirit through the tough times.

ATTITUDE

We hear these all the time: Accentuate the positive, eliminate the negative. The power of positive thinking. Look at the bright side.

How, someone might ask, can anyone remain cheerful and optimistic when he or she has cancer and is going through a debilitating therapy? Obviously, this is an unenviable situation for which no one would wish. But there *are* two sides to everything. Is the glass half-empty or half-full? Of course it is both—but which way you choose to emphasize makes a big difference in how well you tolerate chemo.

Many patients and many health care workers have found that a positive attitude—toward chemotherapy, their chemotherapists, and life in general—helps people cope better. Those who are highly motivated and do not let chemo get them down, who strive to assume as normal a life as possible, who remain actively involved and live their lives to the fullest, who work and play and cultivate hope instead of passivity, inactivity, and despair—these are the people who do best during their time on chemotherapy. This patient's good attitude helped her cope well. "I told my mom, 'It's cancer,' and we both started crying. We cried for about five minutes and then I said, 'Okay that's enough.' I then went on an errand. That's how you have to handle it. You cannot let it monopolize your life. I've seen too many who died because they gave up. And you can't give up."

Rena Blumberg wrote of her experiences during an intensive course of chemotherapy for metastasized breast cancer during which she remained energetic and able to "celebrate" each day. She calls her book *Headstrong*, a word meaning "to have your own way," but which she means in a very positive sense. She writes:

> "For me, 'having my own way' meant I was going to *survive*. To live—and live fully. This took willfulness, to be sure. And at certain moments, particularly during chemo, yes, it took downright obstinacy. But more than any other attitude, I feel this 'headstrong' approach to coping with cancer was the quality that allowed me to survive and to get on with the business of living and living joyously."

However, blind, unquestioning faith or a complete Pollyanna stance may be harmful. You can't always ignore the negative—doing so is unhealthy if it prevents you from taking any corrective action. But by allowing the positive to take precedence you become free and have more energy to take care of the negative.

"A realistic attitude is the key," says Lari Wenzel, former director of the Cancer Information Service at the Comprehensive Cancer Center for the state of Florida:

"Cancer patients in general show a good deal of hope about their future. However, some do feel helpless— that they are not going to respond to treatment, not going to get well, so why bother. Sometimes they don't voice this, but it comes out in their actions. For example, if they are physically able to work, but don't. They may become reclusive, do not see their friends, and shut off their support systems. These patients could benefit greatly from counseling."

Chemotherapy patients should first be convinced that they want the treatment, and second remember that the purpose of chemotherapy is a longer, better life. As Dr. Michael Van Scoy-Mosher, an oncologist at Cedars-Sinai Medical Center in Los Angeles, says, "Patients need to realize that chemotherapy is not the enemy—the cancer is."

COMMUNICATION

The value of telling others about your hopes, fears, needs, and wants is a recurrent theme in the discussions with patients and health care workers and in the literature on coping with cancer. Just talking about your feelings, admitting you have them, can be therapeutic, even if you don't find the exact words to describe them. An open, communicative relationship with your doctor or nurse can be a real advantage and play a central part in how well you do with chemo. But a lack of communication with friends and family is one of the most common and troublesome scenarios of cancer patients. This is often the fault of both the patients and their families and friends, to one degree or another, and is a shame because they all can be the most valuable source of emotional support for each other. It is ironic, then, that poor communication often results out of each's concern and desire to protect the feelings of the other. Although people who are close to each other may be more sensitive to unspoken feelings, they are not clairvoyant. No one can begin to grasp what you are going through unless you tell them. And you cannot expect people to understand and act upon your wishes if you do not give them any clues.

Of course, it is difficult for some people to talk with each other under normal circumstances and the stresses of cancer can accentuate the problem. Lari Wenzel observes:

"There are certain patients who have difficulty addressing their emotions or fears. They may have lived their entire lives in this fashion. Having the diagnosis of cancer will not necessarily lead them toward self-disclosure. For example, men tend to verbally acknowledge their feelings less than women do, probably due to the socialization process. Generally, people who are well-educated about their disease tend to be more acutely aware of their feelings and can discuss them at length."

Dr. Bukberg says she has had people come to her for therapy because they really believed their families couldn't tolerate hearing about their situations. "They really needed to sit down with somebody and talk," she says, "before they could get it together and do the talking that needed to be done with their families."

The severe stress of cancer and chemotherapy can aggravate or accentuate one's style of coping, exacerbate present problems, or bring up old ones. In couples, observes a social worker who has treated many cancer patients, this can create a problem. "Typically, a man may want to cope through action, by doing an activity. The female may want to cope by talking. If that becomes exaggerated—the male wants to distance himself more, the female wants to talk, they may find they have a problem." She continues:

"Sometimes this takes the form of what I call dissynchronization. An example is the forty-year-old man with acute leukemia. He and his wife would sometimes have trouble communicating and used fighting as a way of reengaging with each other; that was their style. When he went back into remission, they were both very relieved, but the rhythm and pacing of their relationship had been thrown off. They found that they were both very distant from each other, very uncomfortable, and unhappy. She was afraid to face the possibility of his death, of fighting with him and being angry with him, and of being open and valid with him because she was so afraid what she might do to him. But also she was fearful of getting reengaged with him and going through the same pain again. But she was able to look at what she was doing and work out another mode of relating. It made marvelous changes in their relationship."

EDUCATION

Often mental states such as fear, anxiety, anger, confusion, and repression are due to a lack of information. Fear of the unknown and an inaccurate picture of reality are two circumstances the chemo patient should guard against. The reality of your situation is tough enough to deal with—why add to it unnecessarily? A well-informed patient usually does better in many ways than an uninformed patient. You only can feel you are in control and make wise decisions if you have the facts and can compare the options. The better you understand your therapy—what its goals are, what the side effects may be, and what can be done about them—the better you will tolerate it, and the less ominous it will seem. It may help to have a clear picture of your prognosis, and to realize that a diagnosis of cancer is not an automatic death sentence: Heart attack victims generally have a much worse prognosis than we do. .

Posing questions to your doctor or nurse is the best place to start getting whatever information you need and want. Write down your questions as you think of them so you don't forget them; take notes or bring a cassette tape recorder. Many patients find that bringing along a clear-thinking friend or relative is a great help—when you're under the kind of stress that cancer imposes it's usually difficult to retain everything you hear.

Dr. William Grace, chief of Oncology at New York's St. Vincent's Hospital, notes that "things go in one ear and out the other. I insist that my patients have notepads. They write everything that I tell them. And then they write down their questions to me, while leaving enough space between them to write the answers. This is a stressful environment, and otherwise, they forget."

Remember: Physicians may sometimes seem to be magicians, but they are never mind readers. They are trained to tell you only the basics and to depend upon you to cue them as to how much further detail to supply. Patients vary greatly in their needs to know and in their abilities to absorb information. So if you want more than you have gotten, you must come out and ask. Don't be shy or feel guilty for taking up your doctor's time. On the other hand, if you want less information—if you can do without the technical details—let the doctor know that too. Too much information, especially when given in a small time span, can be overwhelming and thus just as harmful psychologically as too little information.

Sometimes an outside person such as a social worker can help. Patients sometimes have inner conflicts about the amount of information they want and what it means to them, as this case illustrates:

> "A classic problem is 'The doctor isn't telling me anything.' Well, that may be, but it could also be that the doctor is telling the patients more than they can process. Or maybe they haven't asked the questions.
>
> "I once saw a patient, a young man with advanced cancer who was very sick. He complained that the doctor wasn't telling him how the chemo was working, and he didn't know whether he should keep fighting. I said, 'Have you asked him?' He said, 'Well, no.' I gave him some ideas about questions to ask the doctor, such as 'What would happen if I stopped? What would happen if I stay on the drugs? Would you still take care of me?' He asked me to write them down. He ended up not asking the doctor. In fact, he already knew the answers but was struggling with the conflict inside himself."

If you want to learn more about your cancer and its treatment, you can go beyond your health care providers and turn to booklets, medical journals, and pamphlets. If you are unable to go yourself to the bookstores and libraries, you can ask a friend or relative to do the legwork. This is one concrete way that people can help you and they are usually more than happy to do so, as was the case with this patient:

> "My doctor was very vague about everything—especially my prognosis and the other treatments available. And I wanted to *know* before he began pumping that stuff into me. My friends were very supportive and photocopied articles from medical journals for me to read while I was still in the hospital. It made me feel a lot better knowing what the whole story was."

You may have trouble deciphering some of the medical terms and concepts in the technical or scholarly publications, so perhaps your physician, oncologist, or other doctor will help explain whatever you don't understand. Other sources for information are cancer agencies and societies, and large cancer centers listed in the Sources section.

ASKING FOR HELP

Many chemotherapy patients and their families are very good at coping and can bounce back easily—or they become experts quickly. However, many other patients and their families can use some outside help. This does not mean that they are weak or helpless. It simply means that outside help can make them cope better during a time of extraordinary stress.

It is logical to turn to friends, family, and co-workers for emotional support, and we may be more comfortable expressing our innermost thoughts to those who are close to us. However, this may not always work out or be enough. We may, for one reason or another, get negative reactions. Those people may withdraw: Sometimes the very people to whom we would like to turn are having trouble coping themselves. We may, in fact, feel less comfortable baring our souls to people we know than to people who will be less judgmental, more objective, and who are experienced listeners, counselors, or therapists. Fortunately there are many alternative sources for emotional support, both for ourselves and for our families. We may turn to our doctors or nurses, certainly, but they are often not trained to give emotional support. Social workers, the clergy, support or self-help groups, or patient volunteers are better targets for our outpourings. Or a psychotherapist, family therapist, or a stress-management technique may be what we need.

Of the huge variety of forms of psychosocial support, one or more is bound to be right for you. You might require help for extended periods—all through chemotherapy and possibly thereafter. More commonly, though, patients and their families find that they need a "leg up" only periodically, when some new twist in the situation makes them feel too overwhelmed to cope on their own. (These "twists" may coincide with the crisis points mentioned earlier.)

Dr. Bukberg says that the appropriate help depends upon what the problem is and who the person is:

"A group is a very, very good place to start. If the problem is that you're feeling kind of alone, and going through a rough situation, and other people obviously do not understand in the same way that another person going through it can, if you're feeling very different from other people—and these kinds of things can make you feel so awful—for a lot of people a group is probably the best thing."

Ms. Christ also thinks that "educative/support groups are useful for most patients; most can benefit. Talking with a patient volunteer—someone who has gone through the experience—is also valuable." Too, Dr. Bukberg points out that "the behavioral approach may also be a good first step for people who are having a lot of tension, anxiety, and/or those who are having difficulty with anticipatory nausea. Progressive relaxation, hypnosis, and imaging techniques are appropriate."

When is a support group not enough? Ms. Christ says:

"People might need some help if a patient experiences prolonged sadness and distress. After a period of time of feeling upset or bad physically, people usually are able to have good periods too, when they feel relaxed and a little bit more like themselves. They have moments of being upset, of crying. But if their depression is continuous, some counseling may be helpful."

Dr. Bukberg adds:

"There may come a point where an emotional reaction may be so intense that you want some professional help beyond a support group, even a professionally led one. What those groups are trying to do is provide support—provide the opportunity to help others, get some help oneself, and to feel included in a group instead of feeling outside. They also teach some coping mechanisms, for example, how did someone else deal with a difficult situation?

"But if, after people have tried something like that, anxiety is still really high, or depression is still really bad—if it's interfering with their functioning, if people can't concentrate on work, if their relationships with others around them seem to be disrupted—then it's worth taking a look and trying to see what else may be going on, what else could help. Sometimes counseling that's meant to explore an individual's particular situation can just help clarify things."

Occasionally, psychotherapy can help, according to Dr. Bukberg. "Psychological meanings that a person may not be so much aware of also affect how they are experiencing a stress, and people sometimes find themselves reacting in surprising ways. Psychotherapy can uncover what some of these additional meanings are and sometimes that helps." She gives the example of people whose self-esteem is very tied up in particular parts of their bodies—their breasts or their hair. "The loss of these is obviously much more devastating than it is for people who have other things in their lives that are more important for their self-esteem."

THE CHEMO BLUES

Depression is perhaps the most common and debilitating emotional reaction in chemotherapy patients. At some time or other almost everyone—even the staunchest optimist—feels pessimistic, down, sad, weepy, blah, and blue:

"I'm a very lively person. I'm not a depressed person. But I do get depressed over my illness. I wish I were healthy like everyone else."

"I would be depressed many times. I kind of spaced out, just withdrew. I would cry very easily. I felt so different from the person I had been, the person I knew. I felt like an observer of life because I was so debilitated, so out of it most of the time. And I was so used to being a participant."

As the patients and cancer professionals that speak on the next few pages show, depression is perfectly normal. They also show that the coping mechanisms just discussed can help a great deal to lift you out of your depression and to prevent it from becoming incapacitating or unbearable.

Depression in chemo patients can happen at any time, but it doesn't usually settle in until after some earlier reactive stages have been experienced. Many patients are well into their treatments and have been through all the terrifying, (and to me, exciting) and demanding parts, before the pressing weight of depression becomes noticeable or intolerable. One oncology nurse finds that, for instance, with people on a two-year protocol, "Once they get through the first year and into the second, it's really just awful. But at any midway point patients tend to have a downward feeling—'Are we ever going to get this over with?'"

In my case, the tensions and insults accumulated gradually until one final event provided the crucial jolt. I seemed to be coping just fine until the side effects really kicked in. My oncologist said that the toxicity had finally built up, and I started to feel really sick about one month into the treatment, and really down. And then my hair fell out, which made it even worse. A little while later, John Lennon was killed, and that really did it. Between that and the cancer, I felt as if a part of my past had died, was gone forever, and nothing would ever be as carefree, as good, as it had been before.

Grace Christ explains that depression in chemotherapy patients is usually a "reactive" depression. "Chemo patients are depressed for a good reason," she says, in that they are feeling sad and down as reactions to a specific external event.

Lari Wenzel points out:

> "The conditions surrounding the treatment could promote feelings of depression. If you are feeling physically ill all the time, or a good deal of the time, you are not looking your best, your life has been disrupted, and you know your life is also being threatened, which is why you are undergoing the treatment . . . it's quite easy to understand why people become depressed."

Matthew Loscalzo, a social worker at Memorial Sloan-Kettering, says he sees a lot of depression:

> "There are hundreds of different theories on depression. Some propose it's due to a learned helplessness. We often see this in our patients at Memorial, and I think it's one of the key issues. Another theory is sensory deprivation: People who are not stimulated amply get depressed and tend to withdraw. Cancer patients are physically depleted, with chemical changes taking place because of

the cancer and chemotherapy; their personal space is violated by everyone from the cleaning lady to the doctors, and by everybody else in between. They don't understand what the doctors are saying half the time. And they're not up to snuff—their thinking processes may not be too clear because of the cancer or treatment or both. Patients need to be actively involved in their own care."

In addition, there is some evidence, and some professionals believe, that the drugs themselves cause chemical changes that lead to depression. Mood changes are not unusual when the hormone-producing endocrine system gets thrown out of order. For example:

"After the second treatment, I got a depressed feeling after I got home; I felt very down. The next treatment I got a depressed feeling on the way home. Then I felt it as I got to my car, and became weepy as I drove home. Then it was when I got to the front steps of my doctor's office. By the time of the ninth or tenth treatment, I really went berserk. At the end, I couldn't make it out of his office. What upset me was that I always felt I had been a together person."

"I had terrible mood swings. If you looked at me, I cried. I never knew if it was the surgery, or the drugs, but I was in chemical menopause at that time. And I remember my mother going through menopause and having some tremendous mood swings. She was a real bitch at times; I became a bitch at times. Even I didn't like me. I remember one day I came home from work; I was off the next day. I just locked the door and didn't answer the phone, didn't do anything. I just sat. God, I didn't like myself for a long time! I didn't put on lipstick or take care of my hair. I didn't care what I looked like. Hell, I didn't like me so why should anyone else?"

Depression is bound to go hand in hand with not feeling well for a prolonged period of time. As one patient said, "It just wears you down." So some aspects of depression can be alleviated when physical side effects are taken care of. This book gives many suggestions for relief; perhaps a support group or your oncologist will be able to guide you further or suggest more.

Patients often find that mental or physical activity is an antidote for the blues—sitting around doing nothing but feeling sorry for yourself is not only boring, it encourages you to dwell on your problems. Time could be so much better spent on enjoyable, esteem-building distractions such as hobbies, friends, social functions, work, or support groups. Exercise has many advantages and has gotten many a chemo patient out of the dumps. The fact that they don't feel like themselves does not stop them from doing whatever makes them happy. Some people have let—or have learned how to let—others help keep them cheerful and maintain perspective.

I was at the very bottom of my depression—the pits—when a girlfriend of mine called with some horrifying news. A young man we knew—in his twenties and about to be married—was in an accident and was paralyzed from the neck down. Awful as it was, it really shook me out of my own depression. What the hell was I so upset about compared to his bad luck? At least I could walk, work, do things.

Depression still remains somewhat mysterious. Sometimes no matter what you do, it stays. However, the pros offer their own suggestions for depression. A social worker, for instance, says, "Medication can help; sometimes other things can be helpful. Exercise, biofeedback, relaxation techniques, hypnosis, whatever makes patients feel a little better, helps them to get cognitively out of themselves, to remove themselves from the experience." Mr. Loscalzo has observed that patients feel that "they have no control over the future and they don't know what the future holds. That often makes them feel depressed. Hypnosis is one way to help people feel more in control."

Some recommend strongly psychotherapy or counseling or a support group to help with depression. But Lari Wenzel reminds us that "therapeutic effectiveness depends in part on the patients and their willingness to face and work through the issues surrounding themselves and their illness."

····· CHAPTER 16

The Aftermath

As with most chemo patients, it would be an understatement to say I looked forward to my last treatment. Although chemotherapy wasn't as bad as I thought it would be, I was very glad it was over. After giving me my last injection, my oncologist smiled, shook my hand, and said, "Congratulations. You made it. Now you can go out and play." In spite of the side effects and the misgivings, I had managed to see it through to the end. I felt a real sense of accomplishment. I was free at last! No more nausea; no more fatigue; no more jabbing needles. I *did* go out and play: Michael and I left on a celebratory vacation. I felt high for weeks as I started to look and feel good again; I ate and ate, putting back all the weight I had lost, and then some.

After the first delirious weeks, however, I noticed a strange new feeling creeping in, a vague uneasiness. Playtime was, after all, over. It was time to return to real life. But I had changed; my life had changed. Somehow the old familiar pieces didn't quite fit together the way they used to. I began to realize I couldn't go back to life exactly the way it was. I wondered: What do I do now?

Though certainly happy to be off chemotherapy, many patients experience a similarly bumpy transitional period. This process of "normalization" can be made more difficult by residual side effects, the need for follow-up care, and fear of recurrence. Our old "normal" lives may be beyond out grasp, but we can try to create new "normal" lives for ourselves. To varying degrees, life after chemo will be different, but in certain ways it can be better than life was before. Just as life on chemo is in part what you make it, how you handle the aftermath is up to you.

Dr. Michael Van Scoy-Mosher, an oncologist at Cedars-Sinai Medical Center in Los Angeles, believes that life after chemo is a matter of adaptation. "There's a difference between coping and adapting. Coping, I think, is what you do in an acute situation. Adapting is what you do with a permanent change. In the long run you have to adapt to what has happened to you; it becomes a part of you, it gets incorporated for better or for worse."

Ingrid Bergman, who played two of her most demanding roles (in *Autumn Sonata* and *A Woman Called Golda*) during her eight-year battle with breast cancer, said in an interview that she was determined not to let her illness prevent her from enjoying the remainder of her life. "Cancer victims who don't learn to live with it," she said, "will only destroy what time they have left."

MAKING THE TRANSITION

Once the therapy is over, patients are exhilarated to see side effects subside. Who wouldn't be elated by the return of appetite, strength, and energy, hair growing back, the entire body gradually resuming its normal functions? One patient happily attests: "I was amazed at how quickly I bounced back. About two months after my last treatment, I was running two miles a day again. Unfortunately, I was also expected to cook and take care of the house just like in the old days. But I really didn't mind. It felt good to be me again."

Although this period of normalization is for the most part suffused with relief and joy, it is sometimes tempered by the fact that like any time of transition, it is full of stresses of adaptation for the cancer patient and the family. As side effects diminish, everyone needs to stop thinking of the patient as being sick, to resume former roles and responsibilities, and to start thinking and planning about the future, however uncertain that might be.

Grace Christ of New York's Memorial Sloan-Kettering enumerates some of the psychological and practical difficulties inherent in moving back into the community and normal life:

"There are all kinds of problems and resistances. There may be job problems, insurance problems, problems with confronting an ongoing life, or having to change your goals. Sometimes during treatment you have to constrict your time prespective: You learn to think day-to-day, which is a very useful way to manage a difficult experience. But then you learn to plan ahead, expand your time perspective, make long-range plans, and think more about the future."

After all that activity—treatments, blood tests, side effects, surprises—my life seemed somehow dull, a touch ordinary. So much time and energy had been focused on fighting the cancer, it felt strange to suddenly be doing nothing. I felt like a soldier coming home from active combat: battle weary, but let down by the unexpected absence of danger and excitement.

Sometimes such mixed feelings surface because stopping chemotherapy is anxiety provoking. Much to everyone's—including the patients'—surprise, patients dread or regret the end of therapy because it means leaving the constant surveillance of the hospital, no longer being so closely monitored, and being out on their own. After seeing a doctor every week or two, the security of knowing that if anything develops it will be picked up immediately is suddenly taken away. Some patients do not, in fact, want to go off their chemotherapy and ask their doctors to continue even though it is medically appropriate for them to be taken off it. As one health professional says, patients become so accustomed to doing something to control the illness, that "Being without [chemo] is often really a downer for some people."

"Some people are so relieved that this is not an issue at all," comments Dr. Michael Van Scoy-Mosher. However, he is well aware that patients can have ambivalent feelings about ending the therapy:

"I usually bring up the issue toward the end of the therapy. I'll mention the way some others have felt and try to get my patients to talk about it. Most of the time they have begun to feel that way themselves—I reassure them that they will still be seeing me, not as often perhaps—and discuss the fear of recurrence, and why more therapy is not given. I give them a game plan for follow-up, so although they may not be getting more therapy, they will be closely observed. Beyond that, they just have to cope with it. First they have to cope with getting the therapy, then they have to cope with not getting it.

"I have a patient whose adjuvant therapy I wanted to stop after six months. But she's fought with me to continue it for as long as I can. She's terrified of stopping. It's not as if she doesn't have any side effects, but she's more afraid of the cancer than she is of the side effects. But there are good reasons not to go on with the therapy."

LONG-TERM EFFECTS

Most side effects subside rapidly after treatment is stopped; however, a few may take longer—months or years—and some never disappear completely. There are a few that may even crop up later on. Although these long-term side effects may be annoying or uncomfortable, a few may be debilitating or life threatening. Residual or delayed side effects due to chemotherapy include fertility problems and menopause or menstrual irregularities; hearing, nervous system, liver, heart, lung, bladder, kidney, and blood disorders; diabetes; and second malignancies. In addition, there may have to be psychological adjustments, or patients may need to live with changes due to surgery or radiation. Patients often become very body- or symptom-conscious; so little is known about these long-range side effects that almost anything can be blamed on chemotherapy.

Dr. Charles Vogel, director of the Comprehensive Cancer Center of Miami, admits that "the long-term sequelae of cancer and its treatments have only begun to be noted and understood." It may be difficult to determine where psychological trauma ends and physical damage begins, and whether a symptom is in fact due to chemotherapy or is a condition that might have developed anyway. One patient remarks:

"I still have some nausea now and then, but I've gained back all the weight I lost anyway. People tell me how great I look. I almost feel guilty that I still feel tired all the time. People tend to judge too much how you are by how you look. It makes me feel strange because I don't feel as good as they think I look. People may really wonder if you really have been through all this."

Although basically I'm well and functioning at a normal level, it bothers me that no one can say for sure to what extent I've been permanently affected by chemotherapy. The nausea is gone, my hair is thicker than ever, my blood levels are fine, except for my white blood cell count which is slowly but surely creeping back up to an acceptable level. My menstrual cycle has reasserted itself, though with exasperating irregularity. The foot and leg cramps I suffered during vincristine withdrawal are becoming less frequent, no doubt helped by the advice I got from a physical therapist. These lingering effects, though tangible, are merely annoying, like gnats I can swat away. The one thing the experience has left me with that I find not so easy to handle is a lingering muzziness—a blunting of my physical and mental powers. I often—but not always—feel slightly slowed down, held back. My mind isn't quite as sharp as it used to be, and my energy tends to fade earlier than before. It is subtle, and no one else notices this difference in me, but I feel it is there. Still, this could be an imagined change: Maybe I wasn't really as smart and energetic as I like to think I was; maybe I'm getting older like everybody else; maybe I'm looking for an excuse for real or imagined shortcomings. Or my symptoms may be due to something other than the chemo. But as my oncologist told me, the experience does make a dent in you. I still feel "dented" and probably always will to some extent. Although I may never be "good as new," time and effort continue to help straighten things out, and perhaps I'll ultimately end up better than new.

That the adjustments that post-chemo patients need to make are complex, varied, and challenging has only begun to be recognized. One giant step toward understanding and documenting the ramifications of surviving cancer therapy is the two-year-long study begun by Stanford University Hospital in 1981, the purpose of which was to identify the long-term psychosocial and functional effects in Hodgkin's disease survivors. Dr. Richard Hopper, a radiation oncologist, was the principal investigator in the study; the subjects consisted of patients who received either chemotherapy or radiation alone (40 percent) or both (60 percent).

Although as of this writing, the results are still in an early, preliminary form and have not yet been formally published, they do indicate that for cancer survivors it is not simply a matter of taking your medicine and then picking up your life where it left off. Patricia Fobaire, a social worker at Stanford, who was involved with the study, says that it is finding that about 25 to 30 percent of the patient subjects do seem to have lingering loss of energy and depression for years after the treatment is over.

An intriguing overview of the post-chemo patient's plight comes from Ellen L. Maher of the Department of Sociology at Indiana University. She interviewed fourteen cancer survivors and published her findings in 1982. Talks with these patients revealed that although they were in remission or possibly cured, all were not completely at ease with their good fortune. Ms. Maher describes their unease as *anomia*, a mental state characterized by confusion and anxiety, uncertainty, loss of purpose, and a sense of alienation.

Ms. Maher discusses the many factors that contribute to this strange, vague, unexpected discomfort that can occur when chemotherapy is stopped: The patient's initial perception of a poor prognosis and hence an unanticipated cure or remission; a sense of loss of purpose if a great deal of time and energy has gone into the treatment; uncertainty about the advisability of stopping treatment; the possibility of recurrence and its attendant insecurity and anxiety; the inability to make the switch from "living one day at a time" to thinking about future-oriented activities; ambivalent feelings toward the imperfect system to which patients nevertheless owe their lives; and the withdrawal of support from health care givers and families who are convinced that "the healthiest thing is to put it all behind," even though the patient is not quite ready to do so.

As the number of cancer survivors increases every day, clearly more studies along these lines are needed if patients are going to be helped to live their hard-won lives more fully, rather than to just "survive."

SURVIVOR'S SYNDROME

Perhaps the biggest, most frustrating obstacle to enjoying a full, happy post-chemo life is the possibility of having a recurrence. Naturally, anyone who has been treated for cancer is concerned about a recurrence; and when chemotherapy was less effective than it is now, many people did indeed have recurrences, some quite soon after therapy. Some of course, still do, but now that long-term remissions and cures have become more common, a new medical phenomenon has been born: the Survivor's Syndrome. This anxious state of mind has also aptly been dubbed the Damocles Syndrome, after the character in Greek mythology who sat at a banquet under a sword that was precariously suspended by a single hair. We, like Damocles, see that a sword hangs over us and never know how long we have until the hair breaks and the sword drops. A former mastectomy patient expresses this: "Sometimes I'm afraid to look at my other breast. I do self-examination, but I'm afraid I'll find something. I'll cover it up; or I'll take showers in the dark. It's not that I'm ashamed of the mastectomy—I'm afraid of something showing up in the other breast."

The necessity of follow-up care, with its frequent medical checkups and tests, places an additional stress on post-chemo patients, with each serving as a reminder of a time in the past and of a possible future that most patients would prefer not to think about. Sometimes a physical crisis—any new symptom, no matter how minor—sets off an inner alarm:

"Every time I go to the doctor for a follow-up, I am forced to remember why I am going and I think, 'Oh God, will he find anything this time?'"

"My surgeon is very, very thorough when I go for exams. It scares me he's so thorough—you want him to find it if it's there, but you're hoping he doesn't."

"Now I've turned into a very paranoid person. When any little thing goes wrong ... One night I turned over on my stomach, and I felt a soreness in my rib. I kept pushing it and pushing it to see if it still hurt, and of course the more I poked at it the more it did hurt. It was only a month away from my regular time for a bone scan, mammogram, and chest X ray, so my doctor suggested we do it then, just in case, rather than wait.

"My husband came with me and I waited around inside while they looked at the results quickly to see if they had to be done over. The nurse and a doctor came in, and I couldn't wait to ask them how they looked. They said, 'Oh fine, there's nothing abnormal.' I can't tell you how relieved I was ... I heaved a huge sigh and went out to see my husband, who looked at me and didn't know what to do—I broke out into this big smile and all I could say was 'They're okay.' He broke out in such a smile and began to cry. I never realized how frightened he was too. We both sat there—he was hugging me— just crying like a couple of idiots."

Ms. Christ has noticed that people may have strong reactive feelings on their "anniversaries"—the day of surgery, the day of diagnosis, the start or end of treatment. Approaching benchmarks of one, two, five, or ten years can also cause considerable anxiety. In addition, Ms. Christ notes:

"Sometimes normal life phases such as getting married or having children can be difficult for people because they're markers in their lives. They can remind someone who's had cancer of the whole traumatic experience.

"Young people who have had Hodgkin's disease— when do they tell the people that they're dating? What do they say? If they're going to get married, then they have to confront the question of how long their lives will be. Are they going to be able to have children? There are a lot of uncertainties about that. What kind of sexual partners are they going to make? And if they are going to be able to have children—what impact will this have on their children?"

In addition to a recurrence, patients may be concerned about developing a second cancer in the years to come. Although the percentages vary, patients who have had one cancer are statistically at a higher risk of developing additional cancers than is the average person of getting an initial cancer. There are several theories as to why this may be so.

Possibly factors that led to the first malignancy are also responsible for allowing a second to arise and flourish. Regardless of the form of treatment, people who have had certain types of cancers seem to be more prone later to development of other specific types of cancers: Breast cancer is associated with colon cancer, colon cancer with cancer of the endometrium, and uterine cancer with rectal cancer; cancers of the female reproductive system in general tend to occur together with cancers of the digestive and respiratory systems. Those who have had cancer of the breast, ovary, skin, head and neck, bladder, colon, or rectum are at a higher risk of getting another cancer in the same or paired organ. Finally, since heredity seems to play a role in the development of some cancers, there may be worries about other members of the family getting cancer. This issue is especially prominent when a woman with breast cancer has a daughter who it is feared might also get it.

Another group of statistics shows that people who have been treated with chemotherapy and/or radiation are more likely to develop cancer—usually leukemia—later on. This is usually associated with Hodgkin's disease patients and specific drugs that belong to the alkylating group. Whether this is because the treatment has suppressed the immune system or is itself carcinogenic, or both, is not certain.

In general, people tend to either minimize the possibility of a relapse or exaggerate it. Some people think about it almost all the time, others almost never. Although they run the risk of ignoring real problems that could be successfully treated if they were acknowledged early, true minimizers are lucky. They seem to be able to absorb the shock and go on to live full, happy lives. The others, the worriers, seem to be unable to forget their cancer even for a moment. They are obsessed by their disease and their health; they anticipate the worse to such an extent that it taints the remainder of their lives, by overshadowing and taking time away from the more pleasurable and positive pursuits that life has to offer. Dr. Richard Gralla, an oncologist at Memorial Sloan-Kettering, says about this:

> "Part of coping with chemotherapy is being well, being free of disease, doing the normal things, but still have that sword hang over you. Of course it's more real for the post-chemo patient, but that same sword hangs over me. As a human being living in modern society I can get cancer and I have to deal with it too. I can ignore it—as can you—but that's probably not too healthy. I think it's better to come to grips with it rather than totally ignore the issue."

Dr. Van Scoy-Mosher points out that fears of a recurrence generally recede as time goes by. "I find that although this concern never goes away completely it does get better and patients are able to tolerate it. It depends upon their capacity for denial: Some people are defenseless and don't have a capacity for denial—they can't push things back and those are the people for whom it is worse."

Many people believe that the ability to maintain hope is what provides cancer patients with the strength to go on in spite of the sword of their own mortality hanging over them.

Natalie Springarn, a journalist, had been living with cancer for many years when she wrote *Hanging in There*. In her book she eloquently and unflinchingly describes what it is like to be "hanging in there," to live the different life of the subculture of the "not-well." It is tough for her to keep going, but keep going she does, helping herself lose her fear by keeping alive her hope in the future. She writes:

> "Unlike most 'normal' people, we subculture members have to live with the persistent knowledge of our own mortality. 'Background music' Stewart Alsop called that knowledge, and it is true that when I am occupied the fearful dark tones stay in the background. But they can blare forth, affecting my attitude and ability to get on with the business of living. I have found no skill more important (no matter how it's gained) than the ability to believe in my own survival."

The reasons for someone's uncertain health remaining subdued "background music" or becoming a full brass band may vary. The psychiatrist at St. Vincent's Hospital in New York, Judith Bukberg, thinks that "people have certain styles of coping based on who they are. If you've had a life of bad things happening to you, then obviously you're going to have more of those thoughts than somebody who hasn't; similarly, some people are pessimistic by nature." She continues:

> "It's useful for people to know that the Survivor's Syndrome exists, even though it's difficult to give specific solutions. I do think that continuing support groups are very important. So are hypnosis and other kinds of relaxation techniques. If you tend to be anxious about things, and you want to change that tendency, I'd say the best chance to do that is psychotherapy. Sometimes just by decreasing anxiety, obsessional thinking will stop. Sometimes cognitive approaches can help. It's a shame

that more people don't enter psychotherapy if these techniques don't work."

I had had some dark moments while on chemo, but it seemed easy to dismiss them then—it seemed natural to feel anxious about so many things. I buried my feelings because I was sure I could handle them for the duration, and that things would be fine once I was off the therapy and I could put some time between me and the experience. But about two and a half years after I finished chemo I found it was still hard for me to live with intruding thoughts about my disease and worries about my prognosis. I'd be in the middle of something perfectly ordinary—grocery shopping, for instance—and find myself overcome with sadness. I would think, "What if the chemo didn't work?" I'd have to fight to keep back the tears as I fantasized the bleakest scenario; in pain, unable to work or take care of myself, completely miserable. That I was working on this book, immersed in cancer facts and reliving my experiences daily no doubt heightened my awareness and made my anxiety more acute. In a way, I am grateful for that: If my anxiety had stayed at a low level, I might never have decided that enough was enough and sought help from a psychotherapist. She incorporated hypnotherapy into the sessions and I was able to resolve a lot of unfinished business. I must say the therapy allowed me to feel much better, much more relaxed about having had cancer.

FOLLOW-UP CARE

Even though chemical therapy is finished, as cancer patients we will be getting follow-up medical care for the rest of our lives. Checkups and tests will be regularly scheduled, frequently at first and less frequently over the years as we remain well. Though the last thing we may want to do is spend more time in a hospital or waiting room, follow-up care is a useful and necessary part of post-chemo life. It may be anxiety provoking, but it is also reassuring.

For one thing, follow-up care may be able to address any problems with the residual effects of the therapy. Although our minds and bodies have remarkable resiliency and recuperative powers, sometimes medical support can strengthen us and hasten the recuperative process. Your doctors or other health practitioners may also be able to help you with any practical or psychological hurdles you face in living with cancer. If, for instance, you are preoccupied with your body and any symptoms—at one point I thought every cough might mean lung cancer, every bump or pimple was melanoma, every little ache was a metastasis to the bone, every little bit of constipation was bowel obstruction, every headache was cancer spreading to the brain—talking your fears over with your oncologist and getting some facts and assurances might help. You can ask what the likelihood of spread is, where the metastases usually occur in your cancer, and what the symptoms might be.

Additionally, many people, especially women who have undergone mastectomies, have found that acquiring a good prosthesis or having plastic surgery to improve their functioning and appearance after surgery is an invaluable coping device. This can be particularly important to the psychological well-being and reconstruction can finally allow people to feel "whole" or "normal" again. Mine has certainly improved the quality of my life from both an emotional and practical point of view.

But regular contact with your oncologist is perhaps most advisable because as with primary cancer, the earlier recurrent cancer is detected and treated, the better. As we have seen, cancer is not an automatic death sentence; neither is a recurrence. If you suspect your cancer has spread, do not delay going to your oncologist. Make sure it *is* a recurrence. Get a physical confirmation—blood tests, X rays, and scans. Consider a second opinion. Diagnosis can be inaccurate at any stage of this disease. There are many cases where a patient was presumed to have a metastasis and treated as if he or she was terminal, but was in fact found to be metastasis-free later on.

If there's a recurrence, it may make even more sense than before to turn to psychological support to help deal with feelings of shock, anger, and disbelief; with fears of pain, disability and death, and physical and psychological inadequacies. Patients may find themselves blaming themselves or their families, or feeling betrayed by their bodies and their doctors. Bitterness and a mistrust of the medical system are not unusual. A mental health worker speaks about her awareness of the devastating impact recurrence can have on patients: "This is a very big crisis for people, who kind of thought they were going to do all right, and they *were* all right for a while, and then suddenly . . . it's a very big crisis for the staff too."

As before, be aware of your treatment options. There is usually some form of treatment available, be it standard or investigational. Radiation if often used effectively at this point to reduce pain from metastases; in some cases surgical removal of metastases is successful and justified. It is important for patients to have realistic expectations: Usually no more than a temporary halt to the progression of cancer and/or the palliation of symptoms can be expected when chemo is being used for a second or third time. However, even though additional treatment usually does not offer the chance for a cure, it still may prolong life significantly and can make it more comfortable.

Dr. William Grace at New York's St. Vincent's Hospital, for example, says:

"Sometimes oncologists just run out of therapeutic options and don't have access to newer drugs and methodologies. So it may be fruitful to explore investigational drugs, treatments, and combinations at larger cancer care facilities. Even old drugs may be administered so they are effective. I had a patient with breast cancer who had been through all the medications. We finally decided to give her a drug that had no longer worked for her, and we used it in a new way, called continuous infusion. She had a marvelous response.

"So there are always things to do, although we don't always know exactly what to do in every case. The problem is the combinations and permutations of different cancers, their different sensitivities, the different types of agents—the variables are astronomical. You just do the best you can. If you're lucky, you pull the ace out of the deck."

It is especially important to weigh the cost versus the benefits of treatment for recurrent cancer because the primary goal is to keep patients free of pain and as productive and able to enjoy life as possible. If the side effects are too severe, the quality of life is not being improved. Some people feel that once is enough; having been there, they feel they know what is in store and are reluctant to go through it again.

It is especially important for a patient with progressive disease to have a good relationship with an oncologist capable of seeing patients through the tough times that lie ahead. As always, patients have the right to a second opinion or to refuse or stop toxic treatment altogether.

For some patients, unorthodox treatments may seem more attractive at this point than at the time of original diagnosis and therapy. Many feel that if conventional medical treatment has little or nothing to offer it may be better to pursue an alternate therapy because it keeps their hopes and sense of control alive. Although some alternative therapies are very rigorous and the cost-benefit ratio may be high, many do opt to have them. The Appendix has sources of information about alternative cancer therapies. In addition, there are many books on the subject; *The Cancer Survivors* by Judith Glassman is the best: a thoroughly researched examination of dozens of people who turned to other therapies when conventional medicine offered very little hope.

Even if all therapies fail or become inappropriate and the end draws near, patients should be aware that they can still try to maintain a degree of control over their lives. There is still reason to hope—that the rest of our lives will be as full of dignity and comfort as possible for us and our loved ones. Within the last decade or so, real strides have been made in understanding and coping with this final phase of life. The works of Elisabeth Kubler-Ross and the hospice movements may prove enlightening and comforting, and they are listed in the Appendix.

A BETTER LIFE

Happily, for many of us, a recurrence lies far in the future, or may never happen at all. Whatever time we have left—be it months, years, or a full lifetime—it can be high quality time if we let it.

Many patients have discovered that just because life is different that doesn't mean it has to be worse. Life after chemo can be an improvement over life before. Although shaken, they emerge from the cancer/chemotherapy experience strengthened, with a fresh perspective and a heightened appreciation for the big and little things in life that they used to take for granted, and that others still do. Although the experience may have imposed its share of difficulties, they find it has made them learn about themselves, about others, and about how precious life is. They have learned that the extent to which they can take control over their lives and the way they feel is greater than they ever imagined. Although they may look back wistfully at a more innocent time, they realize one can't go back, one can go only forward, toward a life that may not be normal, but may be better than normal in many ways. Ask them their philosophy and they might tell you, "When life hands you a lemon, make lemonade."

In fact, it seems that these people—those who are able to pull something positive out of having had cancer and chemotherapy—*are* able to cope better. It is important for them to feel that it wasn't all for nothing, that it wasn't all bad. Dr. Van Scoy-Mosher has found this to be true in his practice:

"I've noticed again and again from personal observation that people who seem to cope better than others are able to extract something positive from their experiences. It may be a change in their value systems, their motivations, their family structures, their interests. It may be writing a book about chemotherapy. Often levels of intimacy in a family that were good before are intensified. Even the motivation to adopt a healthier life-style—to stop smoking, to be more careful about your diet—is a good thing."

Dr. Richard Gralla has witnessed this same phenomenon:

"A young patient of mine was on chemo for Hodgkin's. He said, 'You know, as much as I hated the whole horrible experience, it's been about the most important and maturing experience in my life, and it's made a better person of me.' In almost every aspect, from athletics which were important to this fellow, to his life with his wife, to his career, it's made a not very mature adult into a quite mature, quite introspective, and thinking young adult."

The ways people find to express this change are varied. Many choose, for example, to make changes in their diets and life-styles. Some post-chemo patients react by plunging into a kind of live-for-today hedonism and deny themselves no pleasure; others swing in the other direction and adopt stringent dietary regimens in the hope that it will increase their chance for a cure. Still others make no changes. Most, however probably fall somewhere in the middle.

Making constructive, health-building changes can be a very useful, positive step: Becoming involved in creating better health has many benefits, some directly related to cancer. It improves the quality of your life because you feel better, have more energy, and are able to fight illness of all kinds. When you are a participant in positive health building, you help reduce some of the anxiety and let-down about stopping chemotherapy or any active medical treatment. Optimizing the strength of your immune system and all your organ systems may be able to inhibit the growth of any residual cancer or secondary cancer. This is a very important possible benefit, given the fact that we are at such high-risk. Additionally, the healthier you are, the better you will be able to cope with a relapse, should one occur.

My oncologist believes that "what one does after chemotherapy needs to be individualized," just as in the case with what one does while on chemo. He stresses common sense and moderation:

> "Obviously one doesn't get into the situation where one is going to be tantalizing the system anymore than is necessary. Does a person go out and smoke cigarettes because now he or she is as free as a bird? No, that would be foolish—nicotine is an immune suppressant. Does one go out and drink barrels of coffee? I don't think so, coffee is a growth stimulant. But does one say that one will never drink a cup of coffee? No, that's not human.
>
> "I think it makes sense to do the things that are the least likely to create second malignancies, since the incidence of second malignancies is high in people who have had one. For instance, it's important to have a fairly high fiber diet that's going to include plenty of good things. Modest intake of vitamins is a good idea. Being involved with things that are life building is a good idea, and getting back into the mainstream is terribly important."

Because the evidence linking diet, stress, and exercise with overall health (and cancer) is building every day, I have made several changes in the way I live. I have reduced my intake of fats and refined carbohydrates and have increased my intake of fiber. I keep potentially harmful chemicals to a minimum and continue to take the vitamin-mineral supplements recommended to me while I was on chemo. I make a continual effort to improve the way I handle stress, and I exercise almost daily. There are no guarantees, but these practices don't compromise my quality of life; they enhance it. Not only do they support good general health (how ironic it would be to beat cancer and succumb early to some other disease I could have easily prevented), they may have direct bearing on my chances of avoiding a recurrence or another cancer. I can't be on chemo all my life, but I can continue in a life-style that the chemo left behind, as well as any new ones that might be produced.

Patients notice and cultivate spiritual and intellectual differences in the post-chemo life too. Natalie Springarn found that having cancer can be a challenge that forces people to grow and search for personal meaning, to set priorities, to view life more critically and intensively, to sort out the things they really want to do and do their best to do them. The prospect of death, she says, can teach you what life is all about. These patients agree:

> "I don't think my life will ever be the same. But that's not a bad thing. It's not even the cancer at this point. It's just the idea—this brush with death—I look at life now and I see how tenuous it is, how very short it is. You have only your moment. Not just me, but all of life. Most of the time you don't recognize how insignificant your life is, or how short. After something like this, you realize that nothing is forever."

> "A couple of good things came out of this whole mess. My relationship with my husband is even better than it had been. People are more important. Relationships are more important. Things that people do that would bother me before, don't bother me anymore. I think about something, 'Is this worth the time and energy?' Things get put in their proper perspective when you're faced with something like cancer."

Since my diagnosis and treatment, the quality of my life and the way I look at things has changed in many ways. I have learned to be more assertive, to ask questions. I have learned to be less accepting of the way some things are, and more accepting of others. A former perfectionist, I've become more tolerant of my failings—and therefore of other people's too. Reaching out and helping others has given meaning to my experience—that's why I wrote this book and speak to cancer groups and individual patients. I have learned how to sit still— every moment, though precious, does not have to be jam-packed with activity; some moments it's okay just to "be," to merely enjoy the fact of existence. Michael has changed and matured too; I am happy to report that our relationship has deepened to the point where we decided to get married six months after my chemotherapy was over.

Many cancer patients find meaning and purpose in their experience by voluntarily sharing it with other cancer patients:

> "People ask me, 'How can you be doing this? Doesn't it bother you to be constantly reminded of old memories?' I say it doesn't really, that I was in their position once— I didn't have anybody to talk to. If I can pass something on, I feel good inside; talking to them is soothing to me too. Out of the nineteen years I've been nursing, the three that I've been counseling cancer patients have been the most rewarding. I was looking for a reason why this happened to me—now I kind of have an idea why it did. If you can just get to somebody—if I can just reach one in five—if they're happy and can adjust to their lives, it can make it all worthwhile."

There are many opportunities to volunteer your knowledge and insights to people who are going through cancer and chemotherapy. Your local hospital, chapters of the American Cancer Society, and the other support groups listed in the back of this book will be able to guide you in finding a situation that is satisfying and helpful to both you and the uninformed patients who need you. You can let your oncologist and friends know that you are available to talk with newly diagnosed cancer patients. Some people prefer to make financial contributions to cancer foundations, or help raise funds for cancer care and research. One woman with malignant melanoma started a newsletter; many others have started local self-help groups. We can always do our bit to publicize cancer and chemotherapy issues—perhaps to help end the mystery and misconceptions that surround this disease and its treatment. We can educate ourselves about cancer prevention and pass that knowledge on to others. Many people find it liberating and therapeutic to talk openly with friends or in front of small groups, or to write an article for the local newspaper or club newsletter. The more people we reach, the easier the path will be for everyone.

No matter how it is expressed, the positive changes that many post-chemo patients have made signify an affirmation of life and a commitment toward improving and maintaining their health and happiness. Death has tapped them on the shoulder and they have said "Not yet," first by taking chemotherapy, and then by continuing to do everything in their power to continue to improve their prognosis and quality of life. They want to give themselves every chance there is by making positive changes in their life-styles, attitudes, and priorities. Whether these include improving their diets, avoiding known harmful substances such as tobacco, getting more exercise, reducing and managing stress, dealing openly and honestly with their emotions, relaxing and enjoying hobbies and friends, having fun, getting rest and sleep, helping others, being productive and enjoying sexual expression, rather than wasting time and energy worrying about things they can't control, they prefer to deal with the things they *can* control.

Many cancer patients are able to make some of these moves toward living better lives while they are on chemotherapy. (See Chapters 6–9.) Those for whom it was too difficult to initiate and maintain such changes: It is not too late now to turn over a new leaf! Whether you have chemotherapy only once or it becomes an intermittent part of your continuing care, you can still live life to the fullest while continuing a multifaceted program to stay in the best possible health.

Dr. Michael Van Scoy-Mosher ended my interview with him with these encouraging words we can all live by:

"There are two components of health. One consists of the aspects that we have some control over; the other of things we don't, like genetics or things that just happen. And I think we have a certain responsibility to at least control what we can. It's not going to answer it all, but I for one, don't want to lie on my death bed and say that I could have delayed death or avoided it but I didn't because of certain things I did or didn't do. With chemotherapy, you have to resolve the conflict of the intellectual side—understanding the need for treatment—

and the emotional aversion to it, in favor of rational thought. You just have to know in your heart of hearts that you did what you could. And you should see that as a source of pride, that you were able to understand it, cope with it, tolerate it, and get it done with. Even though we know it's no guarantee, at least you know you did all you could do."

It took some time and the writing of this book to realize it fully, but I *am* proud I underwent chemotherapy. Though I have mixed feelings about it, I have no regrets. Chemotherapy is not an easy undertaking, no matter how you look at it. It has its ups and downs, its imperfections and uncertainties. But it is too often thought of in solely negative terms. Chemotherapy, when given well, can do a lot of good; this often goes unrecognized or is lost sight of. Yes, I experienced side effects while on chemotherapy, and some have yet to subside completely. But chemo was worth it, and this is true whether it ultimately has given me only a few extra years or a normal life span. Because of chemo, I at least have a better chance of survival; I'm also a different person, a better person, a more knowledgeable person. I walk around during the day and go to sleep at night knowing I gave cancer my best shot. I hope I have helped you to give it your best shot too, and to make your best even better. And that is all anyone can ask.

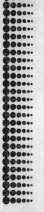

Appendices

Guide to Anticancer Drugs

As we have seen, anticancer drugs (or antineoplastic drugs) kill cancer cells by interfering with their ability to grow and reproduce. They do this either by blocking the cells' supply of essential building blocks for growth or by interrupting the reproductive cycle. Anticancer drugs fall into five main categories, depending upon the way in which they work.

TYPES OF DRUGS

Alkylating agents. These are the oldest chemotherapeutic chemicals we have. These compounds cross-link with DNA—they grab the strands of DNA which then cannot pull apart during cell division. When the cell tries to divide, it self-destructs.

Antimetabolites. These work because they resemble substances that the cell needs in order to grow. The cell mistakes an antimetabolite for the needed substance, absorbs it, and tries to use it during division and growth. Because antimetabolites are not really usable, the cell dies. Drugs belonging to this group were the first to be designed specifically to combat cancer.

Vinca alkaloids. This is a very small, specialized category of drugs that are derived from plant sources. They destroy cells by halting a particular mechanism (mitosis) necessary for the physical process of division.

Antibiotics. Similar to the antibiotics used against bacterial infections, these are derived from naturally occurring soil fungi. They are believed to act by blocking cell growth through slipping between the strands of DNA and thus preventing it from copying itself.

Hormones. As discussed on pages 14–15, these are naturally occurring substances in the body that somehow either encourage or inhibit tumor growth in some cancers. Synthetic hormones or drugs that suppress the body's production of natural hormones are added during chemotherapy.

Miscellaneous drugs. These include a few drugs such as asparaginase, dacarbazine, and cisplatin, that act in a variety of ways against cancer and don't fit into any of the above categories.

Experience with these drugs has shown that some cancers respond well to a single drug (single agent chemotherapy); these include some chronic leukemias and some lymphomas. Most cancers, however, respond much better when several drugs are used (combination chemotherapy). From the approximately one hundred standard and investigational drugs available, oncologists choose two, three, four, five, or six drugs—and sometimes as many as a total of twelve—to be given concurrently or in a certain sequence. Most protocols are comprised of at least three drugs, which can triple or even quadruple single agent response rates while minimizing toxicity. This is possible because:

· The drugs used have different mechanisms of action so various phases of growth are affected.

· Using several drugs reduces the likelihood of drug resistance.

· The drugs are chosen to work synergistically, with one enhancing the effect of the other.

• The drugs are chosen to produce different kinds of toxicity at different times so the harm to the tumor remains high without increasing the harm to the cells in any one organ or system.

• The dosages are timed far enough apart so the normal cells have time to recover, but the cancer cells don't.

STANDARD DRUGS AND THEIR SIDE EFFECTS

In addition to their desired effects, chemotherapy drugs have unwanted side effects. The list that follows gives the standard anticancer drugs along with their known possible side effects. As you look up the drugs in your treatment plan, remember that these are the side effects that *might* happen—not the ones that necessarily *will* happen. It is highly unlikely that you will experience all or even most of them. A few side effects are not listed because they are so unusual that they occur in only a handful of the people taking the drug. (It is also possible for a drug taken in combination with others to produce other side effects than those when it is taken alone.) In most drugs, the rare side effects far outnumber the common side effects. Whatever the potential side effects of the drugs you are taking, a skillful, caring oncologist will be able to avert or minimize the risks. There are many measures that both you and your doctor can take to prevent most side effects and make others more tolerable.

If you want more information about your drugs and their side effects, ask your doctor, nurse, or pharmacist. Many hospitals are starting to make available to their patients individual drug information cards which list the major common side effects and ways to alleviate them. The package insert that comes with the drug is very informative; in addition, there are several reference books with detailed information on anticancer and other drugs. The *Physician's Desk Reference* (*PDR*) has been a standard source for drug information, but its text can be hard for the average person to decipher. Alternatively there is the *United States Pharmacopeial Dispensing Information* (*USP DI*), published by the United States Pharmacopeial Convention, or its *Physicians' and Pharmacists' Guide to Your Medicines*, which is written for a general audience. *Professional Guide to*

Drugs is another readable source. Your doctor, pharmacy, library, or bookstore are possible sources for these materials. If you are taking investigational drugs, the known side effects will be listed on the informed consent form that you sign before beginning therapy.

Name of Drug	More Common Side Effects	Less Common or Rare Side Effects
Actinomycin-D *see* Dactinomycin		
Adriamycin *see* Doxorubicin		
Adrucil *see* 5-Fluorourocil		
Alkeran *see* Melphalan		
ARA-C *see* Cytarabine		
Asparaginase	abdominal pain nausea, vomiting skin rash, itching difficulty breathing joint pain lightheadedness slow blood clotting liver problems headache irritability loss of appetite weight loss	diabetes risk of infection shaky body movements mouth sores mental depression drowsiness, confusion hallucinations nervousness tiredness
BCNU *see* Carmustine		
Blenoxane *see* Bleomycin		
Bleomycin	fever, chills cough breathing problems skin rash, discoloration	nausea, vomiting fainting hair loss mental confusion loss of appetite change in taste perception

Name of Drug	More Common Side Effects	Less Common or Rare Side Effects
		swollen, painful legs or fingers
		headache
		changes in fingernails
Busulfan	slow blood clotting	lung problems, cough
	risk of infection	skin darkening, acne
	tiredness	loss of appetite
		hair loss
		dizziness, fatigue
		impotence
		nausea, vomiting
		menstrual irregularities
		mental confusion
		breast enlargement (men)
		stomach pain
		joint pain, swollen feet
Carmustine (nitrosourea)	nausea, vomiting	lung problems, cough
	risk of infection	liver problems
	slow blood clotting	loss of appetite
		pain at infusion site
		mouth sores
		tiredness, weakness
		diarrhea
		hair loss
		skin rash, itching
CCNU *see* Cisplatin		
CDDP *see* Cisplatin		
Chlorambucil (nitrogen mustard)	slow blood clotting	hair loss
	risk of infection	nausea, vomiting
	tiredness	stomach pains
		skin rash, itching
		lung problems, cough
		menstrual irregularities
		joint pain, swollen feet
		mouth sores

Name of Drug	More Common Side Effects	Less Common or Rare Side Effects
Cisplatin	nausea, vomiting hearing problems sore throat diarrhea stomach pains risk of infection joint pain, swollen feet slow blood clotting	tiredness kidney problems loss of appetite loss of taste perception numbness/tingling in fingers or toes tremors rapid heartbeat
Cisplatinum *see* Cisplatin		
Cosmegen *see* Dactinomycin		
Cyclophosphamide (nitrogen mustard)	nausea, vomiting loss of appetite menstrual irregularities risk of infection hair loss	tiredness cough painful urination bloody urine liver problems joint pain, swollen feet rapid heartbeat slow blood clotting dizziness, confusion stomach pain skin darkening, flushing headache mouth sores sterility
Cytarabine	nausea, vomiting tiredness, weakness risk of infection slow blood clotting fainting headache irregular heartbeat	stomach pain liver problems mouth sores joint pain, swollen feet diarrhea skin rash
Cytosar-U *see* Cytarabine		
Cytoxan *see* Cyclophosphamide		

Name of Drug	More Common Side Effects	Less Common or Rare Side Effects
Decarbazine	nausea, vomiting loss of appetite redness, pain at injection site risk of infection slow blood clotting	blurred vision confusion, uneasiness headache hair loss joint/muscle pain
Dactinomycin	nausea, vomiting tiredness vein inflammation at IV site risk of infection slow blood clotting	hair loss stomach pain mouth sores skin rash, discoloration, acnelike condition loss of appetite
Daunomycin *see* Daunorubicin		
Daunorubicin	nausea, vomiting hair loss risk of infection shortness of breath	stomach pain heart problems mouth and throat sores diarrhea loss of appetite skin darkening joint pain pain at injection site red urine (not bloody) slow blood clotting
Doxorubicin	nausea, vomiting risk of infection mouth sores shortness of breath hair loss slow blood clotting	stomach pain diarrhea swollen feet, joint pain red urine (not bloody) pain at injection site skin and nail darkening liver problems heart problems
DTIC *see* Dacarbazine		
ELSPAR *see* Asparaginase		
Endoxan *see* Cyclophosphamide		

Name of Drug	More Common Side Effects	Less Common or Rare Side Effects
Epipodophyllotoxin see VP-16		
Etoposide see VP-16		
Floxuridine	nausea, vomiting diarrhea stomach cramps, pain mouth sores	risk of infection vertigo slow blood clotting skin rash, sores depression, lethargy
5-Fluorouracil	nausea and vomiting diarrhea	risk of infection hair loss mouth sores skin darkening skin rash nail problems weakness and clumsiness
5-FU see 5-Fluorouracil		
Hydrea see Hydroxyurea		
Hydroxyurea	nausea, vomiting risk of infection slow blood clotting	diarrhea mouth sores skin rash skin darkening drowsiness, dizziness loss of appetite constipation
L-asparaginase see Asparaginase		
Leukeran see Chlorambucil		
Lomustine (nitrosourea)	nausea, vomiting risk of infection slow blood clotting loss of appetite	tiredness, weakness hair loss mouth sores kidney problems confusion skin darkening skin rash

Name of Drug	More Common Side Effects	Less Common or Rare Side Effects
L-PAM *see* Melphalan		
L-Spar *see* Asparaginase		
Matulane *see* Procarbazine		
Mechlorethamine (nitrogen mustard)	nausea and vomiting risk of infection slow blood clotting menstrual irregularities metallic taste	loss of appetite hair loss hearing problems pain/redness at injection site dizziness, drowsiness headache weakness
Melphalan (nitrogen mustard)	nausea and vomiting risk of infection slow blood clotting	loss of appetite stomach pain joint pain mouth sores hair loss
6-Mercaptopurine	nausea and vomiting risk of infection slow blood clotting	stomach pain loss of appetite mouth sores weakness skin rash liver problems headache dizziness, drowsiness
Methotrexate	nausea, vomiting diarrhea loss of appetite mouth sores stomach pain risk of infection slow blood clotting	hair loss headache liver problems joint pain acne skin rash or darkening shortness of breath, cough tiredness, weakness bloody or dark urine blurred vision
Mithracin *see* Mithramycin		

Name of Drug	More Common Side Effects	Less Common or Rare Side Effects
Mithramycin	nausea and vomiting diarrhea mouth sores loss of appetite	drowsiness fever headache tiredness, weakness slow blood clotting depression
Mitomycin	nausea and vomiting pain at IV site risk of infection slow blood clotting	blood in urine loss of appetite mouth sores hair loss skin rash tingling skin, fingers, and/or toes
Mitotane	nausea and vomiting diarrhea	mental depression drowsiness, dizziness tiredness aching or twitching muscle loss of appetite skin rash or darkening fever visual problems

6-MP
  see 6-Mercaptopu-
  rine		

Mustargen *see* Mechlorethamin		
Mutamycin *see* Mitomycin		
Myleran *see* Busulfan		
Oncovin *see* Vincristine		
Platinol *see* Cisplatin		
Procarbazine	nausea and vomiting diarrhea slow blood clotting risk of infection	mental depression muscle twitching mouth sores skin rash, itching,

Name of Drug	More Common Side Effects	Less Common or Rare Side Effects
	tiredness, weakeness cough, shortness of breath drowsiness muscle or joint pain	darkening nervousness, insomnia nightmares hallucinations confusion, clumsiness headache hair loss constipation tingling or numbness in fingers or toes
Purinethol *see* Mercaptopurine		
Rubidomycin *see* Daunomycin		
Streptozocin	nausea and vomiting pain at IV site	kidney, liver, and blood problems
6-TG *see* 6-Thioguanine		
6-Thioguanine	nausea and vomiting diarrhea risk of infection slow blood clotting	stomach pain skin rash liver problems loss of appetite mouth sores joint pain
Thiotepa	nausea and vomiting pain at IV site risk of infection slow blood clotting	stomach pain loss of appetite menstrual irregularities low sperm counts skin rash headache hair loss dizziness tightness of throat
Triethylene- thiophosphoramide *see* Thiotepa		
TSPA *see* Thiotepa		

Name of Drug	More Common Side Effects	Less Common or Rare Side Effects
Velban		
see Vinblastine		
Vinblastine	nausea and vomiting pain at IV site if drug leaks risk of infection hair loss	headache jaw pain mouth sores constipation mental depression tingling and numbness of fingers and toes muscle pain, weakness loss of reflexes loss of appetite stomach pain low sperm counts skin rash
Vincristine	pain at IV site if drug leaks constipation difficulty walking hair loss headache jaw pain joint pain tingling and numbness in fingers and toes weakness	confusion, agitation dizziness hallucinations depression, insomnia loss of reflexes bloating diarrhea skin rash loss of appetite mouth sores
VP-16	nausea and vomiting	low blood count hair loss headache, fever
Zanosar		
see Streptozocin		

HORMONES AND ANTIHORMONES

Hormone treatment is used mostly in cancers of the reproductive system such as breast and prostate cancer. In many cancers the adrenocorticoids are widely used in addition to anti-cancer drugs because of their ability to help patients tolerate the therapy better.

Name of Medication	Side Effects
Adrenocorticoids (cortisonelike) Prednisone Decadron (Hexadrol) Medrol	increased appetite and sense of well-being sleeplessness and agitation fluid retention and weight gain diabetes high blood pressure increased risk of infection acnelike skin condition stomach and intestinal ulcers loss of potassium muscle weakness hirsutism (abnormal hairiness)
Estrogens ("female hormones") DES (diethylstilbes- trol) Stilphostrol Tace Estradiol	nausea, vomiting fluid retention and weight gain swollen, tender breasts headache, dizziness, depression, lethargy lowered blood calcium heart and circulation problems worsening of nearsightedness or astigmatism, difficulty wearing contact lenses abdominal cramps, diarrhea, constipation changes in menstruation loss of potassium vaginal infections, cervical secretions skin changes excess body hair in males: impotence, enlarged breasts
Antiestrogens Tamoxifen (Nolvadex) Nafoxide	transient nausea and vomiting hot flashes loss of appetite vaginal discharge, itching, bleeding headache
Androgens ("male hormones") Halotestin Depo-Testosterone Deca-Durabolin	nausea, vomiting liver problems lowering of voice, skin changes water retention and weight gain changes in libido

Name of Medication	Side Effects
	constipation, diarrhea
	bladder problems, liver problems
	changes in menstruation
	hot flashes
	itchy, burning vagina
	in males: impotence, enlarged breasts, low sperm counts
Progestogens Delalutin Depo-Provera	nausea, vomiting, abdominal cramps dizziness, headache, lethargy, depression heart and circulatory problems changes in menstruation cervical secretions, vaginal infections decreased libido skin rash breast enlargement or tenderness
Teslac	pain and inflammation at injection site
Megace	none reported

HOW NEW ANTICANCER DRUGS ARE DEVELOPED

The Food and Drug Administration (FDA) and its sister organization, the National Cancer Institute (NCI) are jointly responsible for overseeing the testing of new cancer drugs and other treatments. Since 1955, the NCI has supported a program to identify, evaluate, and make available to the public effective anticancer drugs.

There are over thirteen hundred different investigational protocols in the NCI drug development program.

PRECLINICAL SCREENING AND TESTING

A new drug may be truly brand-new and just-discovered, or it may be an analog—a modified version of a drug that has been found effective. Many of the drugs, or compounds, are submitted to the NCI by industry or universities. All new drugs must eventually be tested on humans (clinical trials). But in order to make this testing as justifiable as possible from a humane and economic point of view, scientists try to learn all they can about the drugs by testing them first in the laboratory. It costs about $600,000 just to screen one drug.

Every year, thousands of chemical compounds are screened. Most of them are not effective against cancer, some, however, are effective but are too toxic to be useful. And every once in a while, a drug is found that is effective without being too harmful to consider using in humans. It has been estimated that out of every forty thousand compounds screened, only one is found useful in human cancers.

The screening process begins by testing the drugs on cancer cells to see if they kill them. This may be done either in vitro (in a test tube) or on tumors in mice. If the drugs are found to be active, they are then tested for toxicity in mice. The results of these animal trials give researchers some idea of the side effects as well as the range of safe dosage for humans. This is accomplished by determining the lethal dose in 10 percent of the mice; the equivalent dose is calculated and the drug is ready to go into phase I human trials. At this point the sponsor of the drug—usually the NCI—files an Investigative New Drug application (IND) with the FDA. The application provides information about the drug, the results of the animal trials, and a protocol or detailed outline explaining the plan for testing the drug. The IND is a license to use the drug on humans experimentally.

Phase I

All drugs in this phase are investigational and are being given to humans for the first time. This phase usually involves fifty to two hundred patients with a wide variety of tumors. These are advanced cancer patients who are dying and who usually know it; they have either failed to respond to earlier standard therapies, or they have a type and stage of cancer for which no effective standard treatment exists.

Phase I studies are *toxicity* studies. The primary purposes of this phase are to determine the maximum dose a person can tolerate before severe, unacceptable side effects occur (toxicity); what the side effects are; whether toxicity is reversible; how to schedule treatments; and how the drug is absorbed, used, and excreted by the body. If possible, the therapeutic effects of the drug are observed and recorded. The plan of treatment, or protocol, is arrived at after studying the results of animal trials; in subsequent phase I trials, the results of earlier phase I tests are also considered in designing new protocols. Tests begin with a low dose of the drug; this is increased according to a logical plan as the testing progresses. The initial dosage is administered to a small group of patients; if no toxicity is observed in the first group, the dose may be doubled in the next group; thereafter, doses are increased by specific percentages in subsequent groups of patients until dose-limiting but tolerable toxicity occurs or until clear signs of therapeutic activity occur. Increasing the dose in the same patient is discouraged because delayed toxic effects of the first dose could be mistaken for early toxic effects of subsequent doses. Such a practice could both obscure the results of the study and result in irreversible damage to the patient. Also to protect the patient against delayed toxicity, relatively long intervals between cycles of treatment are recommended—usually at least four weeks. Sometimes pilot studies are conducted much like phase I studies, wherein a new drug is added to an established combination of drugs to see if there are any drug interactions.

At the end of phase I, investigators have enough information to decide whether or not to carry the drug over into phase II studies. It is felt that a lack of antitumor activity at this level is no reason not to test the drug further; the only reason a drug may be dropped is because of severe toxicity. For example, cisplatinum and streptozocin, two drugs that are highly effective in specific tumors, showed early negative testing results. A small number of patients with a variety of cancers were used, and the doses were below those required to elicit a response. These drugs would have been lost if they had been discarded from the testing program prematurely. Even under ideal conditions, if only one or two out of fourteen patients with the same tumor respond to a drug, it could indicate a possible 20 percent response rate, which is cause for no little excitement in chemotherapy.

Phase II

Drugs that show promise in phase I go on to be tested in phase II. All the drugs being tested in phase II are investigational and some may be only two or five years old. By and large, patients in phase II studies are those with advanced cancer and for whom conventional chemotherapy and/or phase II studies did not work. Phase II may not be their only option for treatment: There may be an alternate conventional chemotherapy or an alternate phase III study.

Phase II trails are *efficacy* studies for therapeutic effect. The primary purpose is to determine the drug's activity against specific cancers, and to eliminate drugs that are inactive for a specific cancer, so a variety of cancers must be entered into these trials. There may be up to six hundred patients participating in a phase II study.

The protocols for early phase II studies are based on phase I results and ongoing animal studies. Investigators know some of the side effects and what dose range is safe. This phase is complex in design: The relationships among the dose of the drug, the timing of the drug, the response, and the toxicity are all studied. Therefore, phase II protocols include a wide variety of plans—different doses and schedules—and each permutation must be tested on each tumor type entered in the study, for a fair and accurate comparison.

When the phase II trial is completed, the drug may be discarded due to lack of efficacy, or excessive or intolerable side effects in relation to the therapeutic effects. If the drug approaches or betters the data that exists for standard drugs, the new drug is entered into the phase III studies.

Phase III

Most patients receiving investigational drugs are in phase III studies. Patients who are offered this treatment are those for whom effective standard treatment exists, but for whom phase III drugs might be better. Only patients with the same type of cancer that responded to the drug in phase II studies participate in phase III. And only drugs that are reasonably certain to be either superior to or in the same range of effectiveness of an established therapy, either alone or in combination, are entered into phase III.

Phase III is a *comparison* study. The treatment usually is compared head-to-head with the standard treatment in use for the same cancers. The new treatment may be a single new drug that is being tested alone or it may be a new drug that is being incorporated into an established drug combination to determine whether it increases the effectiveness and/or tolerability of the established regimen. A patient who chooses to participate may be randomized to receive one of several treatment options. One is the conventional treatment—the best established treatment medicine has to offer at that time. The others are the investigational arms of the study. Randomization is a process that occurs at a central office, a method whereby it is left to chance to choose whether a patient is slated for one arm or the other. It exists to eliminate any possible bias from the doctor. Not all drugs in phase III studies are investigational, only the ones in the investigational arm of the study may be. The protocols for phase III trials are based on the findings from phase II. The dosages and schedules that proved most effective are adopted. After accruing and treating hundreds of patients with the same type of cancer, various statistical tools are applied to compare the data to see if there is a significant difference in the effectiveness of the drugs.

If a new drug compares favorably with the standard treatment and has been tested to the satisfaction of the FDA, then a New Drug Application is filed, which gives permission to market the drug.

Special Conditions

Some drugs are classified as Group C drugs; these have clearly shown to be effective against specific tumors, but for some reason have not become available commercially. The NCI will supply these drugs to physicians for the treatment of individual patients who are not on clinical research trials.

●●●●●· SOURCES

SUPPORT SERVICES

Your local hospital is the best place to start looking for support services in your community. Looking in the telephone directory under "Cancer" (in the white pages) and "Social Service Organizations" (in the yellow pages) will also help you find what you need. This last listing includes the national and regional organizations that are the largest and that will be able to refer you to the chapters near you. Either write them or phone—if the current numbers of the national offices and your local chapter aren't in your directory, you can get them through telephone information.

American Cancer Society
777 Third Ave.
New York, NY 10017
(212) 371-2900

Psychological support, physical rehabilitation, patient education and information, transportation to and from treatment, financial counseling, employment assistance, loans equipment, and blood programs. Supplies surgical dressings and medications.

Cancer Information Service (CIS) 1-800-4-CANCER Hawaii: 524-1234 Washington, DC: 636-5700 Alaska: 1-800-638-6070	Toll-free telephone inquiry system. Supplies information about local and regional resources and programs for those interested in psychological, emotional, medical, physical, financial, and employment assistance, support, and education. Publishes printed educational material. Most are affiliated with a comprehensive cancer center.
Office of Cancer Communications National Cancer Institute Bldg. 31, Rm. 1018A Bethesda, MD 20205 (301) 496-9000	Current, accurate cancer information on standard and investigational treatment; nutritional and emotional support.
The Cancer Federation 10932 Magnolia Avenue Box 4271 Riverside, CA 92514 (714) 359-3794	A research organization that provides referrals to therapists for psychological counseling and physicians who use immunotherapy, scholarships for research, and educational materials.
Cancer Hopefuls United for Mutual Support (CHUMS) 3310 Rochambeau Avenue New York, NY 10467 (212) 655-7566	A national self-help organization that includes crisis intervention, information, self-help rap sessions, educational meetings, and a newsletter. Founded by a psychologist.
Cancer Consultation Service 237 Thompson St. New York, NY 10012 (212) 254-5031	Regional resource for informational counseling about prognosis, diagnosis, medication; and for emotional/supportive counseling to help people think through options and emotional, spiritual, and psychological issues.
Candlelighters 123 C St., SE Washington, DC 20003 (202) 544-1696	Over one hundred chapters, for parents of children with cancer; emotional support and education. Publishes newsletter. Toll-free hotline.

Center for Attitudinal Healing
19 Main St.
Tiburon, CA 94920
(415) 435-5022

Established to supplement traditional health care that helps patients with life-threatening illnesses cope by changing their perceptions about illness and its related problems. Groups, programs, books, and tapes are available.

Cancer Care, Inc.,
National Cancer Foundation
1 Park Ave.
New York, NY 10016
(212) 679-5700

Social service agency that provides professional counseling and planning for patients and families. Consultation, education, nursing care, home health care, homemakers and housekeepers, financial assistance.

CanSurmount
American Cancer Society
Colorado Division
1809 East 18th Ave.
Denver, CO 80218
(303) 321-2464

Patient and family education and information.

I Can Cope
American Cancer Society
777 Third Ave.
New York, NY 10017
(212) 371-2900

Education and psychological support for patient and family.

Leukemia Society of
America, Inc.
800 Second Ave.
New York, NY 10017
(212) 573-8484

Referral to local support services. Financial assistance for drugs and lab costs.

Make Today Count
P.O. Box 303
Burlington, IA 52601
(319) 753-6461

Two hundred local chapters of patients and family members. Peer support groups, lectures, and speakers.

National Women's Health
Network
224 Seventh St., SE
Washington, DC 20003
(202) 543-9222

National consumer rights group concerned with women's health needs, including those related to cancer.

People Against Cancer
(PAC)
American Cancer Society
37 S. Wabash Ave.
Chicago, IL 60603
(312) 372-0471

Recovered cancer patients who are telephone volunteers. Emotional support and information; referrals to other sources of support.

Planetree Health Resource
Center
2040 Webster Street
San Francisco, CA 94115
(415) 346-4636

Offers research packets by mail: a general information one for $5.00 or an in-depth packet tailored to specific medical problem for $35. Researchers draw on medical texts and computer data bases as well as on printed material geared toward the general public; both traditional and alternative approaches are covered.

Psychosocial Counseling Service
UCLA—Jonsson Comprehensive
Cancer Center
1100 Glendon Ave.
Suite 844
Los Angeles, CA 90024
(213) 206-6017

Telephone service of trained professionals who counsel cancer patients, family, and friends.

Touch, Coordinator,
Cancer Control Program
University of Alabama
in Birmingham
104 Old Hillman Bldg.
Birmingham, AL 35294
(205) 934-4000

Assistance for cancer patients and families in coping with cancer and its treatment; peer support, education.

United Cancer Council, Inc.
1803 N. Meridian St.
Indianapolis, IN 46202
(317) 923-6490

Education programs, therapy groups; nursing, homemaking, medication, and prostheses.

United Ostomy Association
2001 Beverly Blvd.
Los Angeles, CA 90057
(213) 413-5510

Five hundred nationwide chapters. Information, peer support, new techniques and equipment; insurance plan for members.

FOR TERMINALLY ILL PATIENTS

National Hospice Organization
1901 North Fort Meyer Dr.
Rossalin, VA 22180
(703) 243-5900

Referral to local hospice programs.

The Concern for Dying
250 W. 57th St.
New York, NY 10019
(212) 246-6962

Nonprofit organization that distributes the living will, which records the patient's wishes concerning treatment.

If you would like more information about hospices, refer to: *The Hospice Movement: A Better Way of Caring for the Dying* by Sandol Stoddard (Briarcliff Manor, N.Y.: Stein & Day, 1977); and *Hospice* by Parker Rossman (New York: Fawcett Columbine, 1979).

NONTRADITIONAL CANCER THERAPIES

Sources for information about nontraditional, or unorthodox, treatments are given below.

Cancer Control Society
2043 North Berendo St.
Los Angeles, CA 90027
(213) 663-7801

Foundation for Alternative Cancer Therapies, Ltd. (FACT)
Box HH
Old Chelsea Station
New York, NY 10113
(212) 741-2790
(Note: The Foundation suggests that you call rather than write.)

International Association of Cancer Victors and Friends
7740 Manchester Ave. #110
Playa del Rey, CA 90291
(213) 822-5032

Ruth Yale Long, Ph.D.
Nutrition Education Association, Inc.
P.O. Box 20301
Houston, TX 77025
(713) 665-2946

HELP WITH THE COST
OF CHEMOTHERAPY

The cost of chemo varies tremendously—from a few thousand dollars to hundreds of thousands of dollars. The drugs themselves account for a good portion of the cost: Some are inherently more expensive that others, but the dosages, the frequency and length of treatment, and the facility at which you receive them can also influence the cost. In addition to the drugs, you will be charged for the administration of the drugs, the doctor's time and examination fees, and frequent tests used to monitor your condition. Add to this any hospital charges if you are admitted for chemotherapy or any serious side effects due to chemotherapy—plus any support services that you will require such as additional drugs, nutritional supplements, hairpieces, psychosocial counseling, or home care personnel. Transportation and accommodations for you and/or your companions may also be a part of the total bill.

Some medical insurance policies cover chemotherapy, some don't. Some cover chemotherapy only when administered in a hospital, and not in a private doctor's office. Some cover only a percentage, some cover 100 percent, some only up to a certain amount. Insurance policies do not cover transportation or accommodations, and some may not cover all the support services you need. Whatever is not covered is tax-deductible.

In some cases, the reactions to chemotherapy are so severe that the patients cannot work or cannot work well while having treatment. Some must follow a reduced work schedule or work performance suffers, or prejudice and fear cause the loss of a job. Even with medical insurance and sometimes even in spite of disability insurance, chemotherapy can be a very heavy financial burden to bear.

You can begin to cope with your financial concerns by discussing them openly with your doctor, nurse, social worker, or health insurance representative. Find out exactly what your insurance covers and how to get maximum coverage. Reading the fine print may reveal that your policy covers chemotherapy only when administered in a hospital, not in your doctor's office, and you may want to adjust your treatment plan. Make every effort to continue to work. You may want to discuss the possibility of modifying your therapy so you are less debilitated. Thoroughly utilize any support services or therapies you need to keep you physically and emotionally as strong as possible.

If you have no insurance, or inadequate insurance, there are several ways to get help. For instance, you can ask a social worker about obtaining Medicare or Medicaid or some other form of public assistance to help pay your bills. The American Cancer Society, the Leukemia Society of America, and Cancer Care, Inc., are examples of sources of financial help with drugs, home care expenses such as housekeepers and nurses, transportation, equipment, and blood transfusions. If you cannot afford chemotherapy, there are many ways to reduce, or at least begin to whittle down, the enormity of the cost.

One patient I spoke to had had several operations, had been misdiagnosed, and was emotionally and financially depleted. She found an oncologist who finally got her diagnosis right, and for her inoperable tumor she was put on maintenance chemotherapy which will last the rest of her life. She says: "I wrote to the company who makes my drug and pleaded my case. I said I could no longer afford my cancer. They now send me the drug for free." Her oncologist allowed his fees to accumulate and her to pay him off (very) gradually.

Chemotherapy is available at some institutions for free. Veterans Administration Hospitals give free treatments to veterans; Public Health Service Hospitals give free treatments to former Merchant Marines and to native Americans. The National Cancer Institute and some other cancer centers give treatments that are wholly free or partly paid for by the institution. Sometimes, but not always, the treatment is experimental. Even if you have financial problems, you will rest easier if you do your homework: Investigate the treatment, the doctor, and the institution to find out if this is a situation in which you feel comfortable.

••••• GLOSSARY

Acute: Occuring suddenly or over a short period of time.

Adjuvant chemotherapy: Anticancer drugs used in combination with either surgery or radiation as part of the initial treatment of cancer, before detectable spread, in order to prevent or delay a recurrence.

Alopecia (al-o-pee'shah): Hair loss, a common side effect of chemotherapy drugs.

Amenorrhea (a-men-o-ree'ah): Abnormal absence or stoppage of menstruation, a side effect of chemotherapy.

Anorexia: Loss of appetitie, a common side effect of chemotherapy.

Antiemetic: A drug used to reduce nausea and vomiting.

Biopsy: Removal and microscopic examination of tissue from the body for purposes of diagnosis. An *exisional* biopsy removes the entire suspicious tissue; an *incisional* biopsy removes only a small portion.

Bone marrow: The spongy inner core of the bone that produces blood cells, usually affected by chemotherapy.

Cachexia (ka-keck'see-ah): The wasting away of the body often seen in advanced cancer.

Cancer: A general term used for over a hundred different diseases characterized by abnormal, uncontrolled cell growth.

Carcinogen: A cancer-causing agent. Carcinogenesis is the causation of cancer.

303

Carcinoma: Cancer that originates in the epithelial tissue (glands, skin, and lining of the internal organs) of the body. Most cancers are carcinomas (80 to 90 percent).

Chemotherapy: The treatment of disease, especially cancer, with chemicals or drugs.

Chronic: Lasting a long time (as opposed to "acute"), said of a condition.

Clinical: Pertaining to direct observation and care of patients, as opposed to research.

Combination chemotherapy: Use of two or more anticancer drugs, together or sequentially.

Complete blood count (CBC): A laboratory procedure that determines the number of red cells, white cells, and platelets in a sample of blood.

Cytology (sy-tol'a-jee): Scientific study of the origin, structure, and functions of cells. Cytotoxic drugs are drugs that inhibit or kill cells in the body, such as anticancer drugs.

Edema (e-dee'mah): An abnormal accumulation of fluid in tissues of the body which causes swelling, a side effect of hormone therapy.

Epidemiology: The study of factors thata influence the frequency and distribution of diseases, such as cancer, in an effort to find the causes and therefore prevent them.

Hormonal therapy: The manipulation of hormone levels in the body which can cause a tumor to stabilize or shrink.

Immunotherapy: An experimental therapy used to stimulate the body's own defense mechanism to control cancer.

Informed consent: A legal standard (put in writing for experimental therapies) that states how much a patient must know about the potential risks and benefits of a therapy before being ale to undergo it knowledgeably.

Investigational New Drug: A drug that has been licensed by the Federal Drug Administration (FDA) for use in clinical trials, but not yet approved by the FDA for commercial marketing.

Lesion (lee'zhun): A change in the structure of part of an organ or tissue due to disease or injury; a tumor is often referred to as a lesion.

Leukopenia: A decrease in the number of white blood cells in the blood.

Lymph nodes: Small, bean-shaped structures in the body that act as filters, collecting bacteria and cancer cells that may travel through the lymphatic system, a part of the immune system. When infection or cancer is present, lymph nodes may become enlarged and are commonly called "swollen glands." Nodal involvement in cancer means that cancer cells have spread from the primary tumor site to nearby nodes.

Malignant: Life threatening in medical terminology it usually means cancerous as opposed to benign.

Metastasis (me-tas'ta-sis): The migration of cancer cells from the primary tumor site to other parts of the body, thereby producing cancer spread. Metastatic cancer occurs when cancer has spread from its original site to one or more distant sites.

Myelosuppression: A decrease in the bone marrow's production of blood cells.

Neoplasm: A new, abnormal growth of cells, also called a tumor, which may be benign or malignant.

Oncologist (on-kol'o-jist): A physician who specializes in cancer. Oncology is the study of tumors, especially cancerous ones.

Palliation (pal'ee-ay-shun): The act of relieving or soothing a symptom, such as pain, without actually curing the cause. Chemotherapy is sometimes used for this purpose.

Pathologist: A doctor who is specially trained to interpret and diagnose the changes in body tissues caused by disease.

Prognosis: The expected or probable outcome of an illness or disease.

Protocol: The outline or plan for experimental treatment, also used for standard treatment.

Recurrence: The return of cancer after its apparently complete disappearance.

Regression: The shrinkage or disappearance of a cancer.

Remission: The decrease or disappearance of detectable disease.

Side effect: A second, unintentional, and usually undesirable effect from a drug or other treatment, besides the primary, therapeutic effect. The primary effect of chemotherapy is to control or kill cancer cells; side effects may be hair loss or nausea.

Single agent chemotherapy: Treatment of cancer using one drug rather than a combination of several drugs.

Thrombocytopenia: A decrease in the number of platelets in the blood.

Titration: A method used to determine the smallest amount of a drug or drugs that is required to bring about a desired effect. In chemotherapy, this balancing keeps the toxicity and side effects to a minimum and the antitumor activity to a maximum.

Toxic: Poisonous.

Tumor: An abnormal mass of tissue that results from excessive cell division and performs no useful function, and which may be benign or malignant.

●●●●●● BIBLIOGRAPHY

Ahmed, Paul, ed. *Living and Dying with Cancer*. New York: Elsevier North Holland, 1981. (Coping strategies)

American Cancer Society. *Cancer Facts and Figures 1983*. New York: American Cancer Society, Updated annually.

Ardell, Donald B. *High Level Wellness: An Alternative to Doctors, Drugs, and Disease*. Emmaus, Pa.: Rodale Press, 1977.

Beattie, Edward J., Jr. *Toward the Conquest of Cancer*. New York: Crown Publishers, 1980.

Begg, Colin B. et al. "Participation of Community Hospitals in Clinical Trials." *New England Journal of Medicine* 6:306 (18) (May 6, 1982): 1076–80.

Bennett, Hal, and Michael Samuels. *Well-Body Book*. New York: Random House, 1973.

Benson, Herbert. *The Relaxation Response*. New York: William Morrow and Company, 1975.

Berkley, George E. *Cancer: How to Prevent It and How to Help Your Doctor Fight It*. Englewood Cliffs, N.J.: Prentice-Hall, 1978.

Blumberg, Rena. *Headstrong*. New York: Crown Publishers, 1982. (Personal account)

Bricklin, Mark. *The Practical Encylopedia of Natural Healing*. Emmaus, Pa.: Rodale Press, 1976.

Brody, Jane. *You Can Fight Cancer and Win*. New York: Quadrangle/ Times Books, 1977.

Bursztajn, Harold et al. *Medical Choices, Medical Chances*. New York: Delta Books/Dell Publishing, 1981.

Carl, William. "Oral Complications in Cancer Patients." *American Family Physician* 27 (2) (February 1983): 161–70.

Christ, Grace H. "A Psychosocial Assessment Framework for Cancer Patients and their Families." *Health and Social Work* 8 (1) (Winter 1983): 57–64.

Cope, Oliver. *The Breast: It's Problems—Benign and Malignant—and How to Deal with Them*. Boston: Houghton Mifflin, 1977.

Cornacchia, Harold J., ed. *Shopping for Health Care*. New York: New American Library, 1982.

Cousins, Norman. *Anatomy of an Illness*. New York: W. W. Norton & Co., 1979.

Cowles, Jane. *Informed Consent*. New York: Coward, McCann & Geoghagan, 1976.

DeVita, Vincent T., Jr. "Progress in Cancer Management." Keynote address to the American Cancer Society National Conference, Washington, D.C., June 24, 1982.

Donoghue, Marguerite et al. *Nutritional Aspects of Cancer Care*. Reston, Va.: Reston Publishing Co., 1982.

Downing, George. *Massage Book*. New York: Random House, 1972. (A classic how-to)

Epstein, Samuel S. *The Politics of Cancer*. San Francisco: Sierra Club Books, 1978. (Environmental carcinogens)

Fiore, Neil A. *The Road Back to Health—Coping with the Emotional Side of Cancer*. New York: Bantam Books, Inc., 1984. (Based on a psychologist's personal and professional experiences.)

Fishman, Joan and Barbara Anrod. *Something's Got to Taste Good: The Cancer Patient's Cookbook*. New York: New American Library, 1981.

Fredericks, Carlton. *Breast Cancer: A Nutritional Approach*. New York: Grosset & Dunlap, 1977.

Glassman, Judith. *The Cancer Survivors—and How They Did It*. New York: The Dial Press, 1983. (Inner and outer resources; alternative therapies)

Glucksberg, Harold, and Jack W. Singer. *Cancer Care: A Personal Guide*. Baltimore: Johns Hopkins University Press, 1980. (With chapters on treatment for specific cancers)

Gold, Michael. "Cancer: When the Chromosome Breaks." *Science 83* 4 (7) (September 1983): 16–17. (Causes of cancer)

Goodfield, June. "Dr. Coley's Toxins." *Science 84* 5, no. 3 (April 1984): 68–73.

Goodhart, Robert S., and Maurice E. Shils. *Modern Nutrition in Health and Disease.* 6th ed. Philadelphia: Lea & Febiger, 1980.

"Guidelines for the Clinical Evaluation of Antineoplastic Drugs." U.S. Department of Health and Human Services Publication no. 81–3112. Rockville, Md.: Bureau of Drugs, Food and Drug Administration, 1981.

Gunther, John. *Death Be Not Proud.* New York: Harper & Row, 1949. (Personal account)

Hanson, P. G., and D. K. Flaherty. "Immunologic Responses to Training in Conditioned Runners." *Clinical Science* 60 (2) (February 1981): 225–28.

Hegsted, D. M. "Optimal Nutrition." *Cancer* 43 (5) (May 1979): 1996–2003.

Hofer, Jack. *Total Massage.* New York: Grosset & Dunlap, 1976.

Hott, Jacqueline Rose. "Restoring Sexual Expression After Uterine Cancer." *The Female Patient* 7 (August 1982): 30/15–18.

Howe, Herbert M. *Do Not Go Gentle.* New York: W. W. Norton & Co., 1981. (Personal account)

Hrushesky, W. M. J. "Circadian Timing of Cancer Chemotherapy." *Science* 228 (April 5, 1985): 73–75.

Inglis, Brian, and Ruth West. *The Alternative Health Guide.* New York: Alfred A. Knopf, 1983.

Intermed Communications, Inc. *Professional Guide to Drugs.* Springhouse, Pa.: Intermed Communications, Inc., 1982.

Kelly, Orville E. *Until Tomorrow Comes.* New York: Everest House, 1979. (Personal account)

Kubler-Ross, Elisabeth. *On Death and Dying.* New York: Macmillan, 1978.

Kushner, Rose. *Alternatives—New Developments in the War on Breast Cancer.* New York: Warner Books, Inc. 1985.

LeShan, Lawrence. *You Can Fight for Your Life: Emotional Factors in the Causation of Cancer.* New York: M. Evans and Company, 1977.

Levitt, Paul M. *The Cancer Reference Book.* New York: Facts of Files, 1983 (Revised).

Lowe, Carl, and James W. Nechas. *Whole Body Healing: Natural Healing with Movements, Exercise, Massage, and Other Drug-Free Methods.* Emmaus, Pa.: Rodale Press, 1983.

Lucien, Israel. *Conquering Cancer.* New York: Vintage/Random House, 1978.

MacDonald, John A. *When Cancer Strikes: A Book for Patients, Family, and Friends.* Englewood Cliffs, N.J.: Prentice-Hall, 1981.

Mahler, Ellen L. "*Anomic Aspects of Recovery from Cancer.*" *Social Science Medicine* 16 (1982): 907–12.

Margie, Joyce Daly. *Nutrition and the Cancer Patient—Resources, References, and Recipes for Coping with Cancer.* Radnor, PA: Chilton Books, 1983.

Maule, W. F., and M. C. Perry. "Management of Chemotherapy-Induced Nausea and Emesis." *American Family Physician* 27 (1) (January 1983): 226–34.

Maxwell, Mary B. "Scalp Tourniquets for Chemotherapy-Induced Alopecia." *American Journal of Nursing* 80 (5) (May 1980): 900–3.

Melluzzo, Paul J., and Eleanor Nealon. *Living with Surgery.* Dayton, Ohio: Contemporary Books, 1979.

———. *Mal(e)practice.* Chicago: Contemporary Books, 1981.

Mindell, Earl. *Earl Mindell's Vitamin Bible.* New York: Warner Books, 1979.

Morgan, Susanne. *Coping with a Hysterectomy.* New York: The Dial Press, 1981.

Morra, Marion, and Eve Potts. *Choices: Realistic Alternatives in Cancer Treatment.* New York: Avon Books, 1980.

Morrow, Gary R., and Christine Morrel. "Behavioral Treatment for the Anticipatory Nausea and Vomiting Induced by Cancer Chemotherapy." *The New England Journal of Medicine* 307 (24) (December 1982): 1476–80.

Moss, Ralph W. *The Cancer Syndrome.* New York: Grove Press, 1980.

National Cancer Institute. *Coping with Cancer: A Resource for the Health Professional.* National Institutes of Health Publication No. 80–2080. Bethesda, Md.: National Institutes of Health, 1980.

———. *National Cancer Program 1982 Director's Report and Annual Plan FY 1984–1988.* National Institutes of Health Publication No. 83–2486. Bethesda, Md.: National Institutes of Health, 1984.

Nierenberg, Judith, and Florence Janovic. *The Hospital Experience: A Complete Guide to Understanding and Participating in Your Own Care.* New York: Bobbs-Merrill, 1978.

Rapaport, Stephen A. *Strike Back at Cancer*. Englewood Cliffs, N.J.: Prentice-Hall, 1978.

Reingold, Carmel Berman. *The Lifelong Anti-Cancer Diet*. New York: New American Library, 1982.

Reitz, Rosetta. *Menopause: A Positive Approach*. Radnor, Pa.: Shilton Book Co., 1977.

Renneker, Mark, and Steven Leib. *Understanding Cancer*. Palo Alto: Bull Publishing, 1979.

Renshaw, Domeena. "How Cancer Patients and Their Families Cope with Cancer." *Medical Opinion* 73 (August 1975): 843–48.

Rogers, Joann Ellison. "Catching the Cancer Strays." *Science 83* 4 (6) (July/August 1983): 42–48.

Rosenbaum, Ernest. *Living with Cancer*. St. Louis: C. V. Mosby Medical Library, 1982.

Rosenbaum, Ernest H., and Isadora R. Rosenbaum. *A Comprehensive Guide for Cancer Patients and Their Families*. Palo Alto: Bull Publishing Co., 1980.

Rosenfeld, Isadore. *Second Opinion: Your Medical Alternatives*. New York: Simon and Schuster, 1981.

Rossman, Parker. *Hospice*. New York: Fawcett Columbine, 1977.

Roth, Jay S. *All About Cancer*. Philadelphia: George F. Stickley Company, 1985.

Rothman, Roger A. *Using Marijuana in the Reduction of Nausea Associated with Chemotherapy*. Seattle: Murray Publishing Company.

Ryan, Cornelius, and Kathryn Morgan Ryan. *A Private Battle*. New York: Simon and Schuster, 1979. (Personal account)

Salsbury, Kathryn H., and Eleanor L. Johnson. *The Indispensable Cancer Handbook*. New York: Seaview Books, 1981.

Sattilaro, Anthony J., with Tom Monte. *Recalled by Life*. Boston: Houghton Mifflin, 1982. (Personal account of cancer treatment with macrobiotic diet)

Scott, Diane W. et al. "The Antiemetic Effect of Clinical Relaxation: Report of an Exploratory Pilot Study." *Journal of Psychosocial Oncology* 1 (1) (Spring 1983): 71–84.

Simonton, Carl O. and Stephanie Matthews-Simonton. *Getting Well Again: A Step-by-Step Guide to Overcoming Cancer*. Los Angeles: J. P. Tarcher, 1978. (Visualization)

Sontag, Susan. *Illness as Metaphor*. New York: Farrar, Straus and Giroux, 1977.

Spingarn, Natalie Davis. *Hanging in There: Living Well on Borrowed Time*. Briarcliff Manor, N.Y.: Stein & Day, 1982. (Personal account)

Stelin, John S. Jr., and Kenneth H. Beach. "Psychological Aspects of Cancer Therapy." *The Journal of the American Medical Association* 197 (July 1966): 28–34.

Stoddard, Standol. *The Hospice Movement: A Better Way of Caring for the Dying*. Vintage/Random House, 1978.

Stoll, Basil A., ed. *Mind and Cancer Prognosis*. New York: John Wiley & Sons, 1979.

Tache, Jean, Hans Selye, and Stacey B. Dan, eds. *Cancer, Stress, and Death*. New York: Plenum Publishing Corp., 1979.

Trounce, J. R. "Antiemetics and Cytotoxic Drugs." *British Medical Journal* 286 (6362) (January 1983): 327–29.

U.S. Congress. Senate. Subcommittee on Investigations and General Oversight of the Committee on Labor and Human Resources. *Examination on Deficiencies in the Use of Experimental Drugs on Cancer Patients*. 97th Cong., 1st Sess., 1981.

U.S. Congress. Senate. Subcommittee on Invesitgation and General Oversight of the Committee on Labor and Human Resources. *Examination of Effective Alternatives Toward Correcting Deficiencies in the Use of Experimental Drugs on Cancer Patients*. 97th Cong., 2d Sess., 1982.

United States Pharmacopeial Convention, Inc. *Physician's Guide to Your Medicines*. New York: Ballantine Books, 1981.

Watson, Rita Esposito, and Robert C. Wallach. *New Choices, New Chances: A Woman's Guide to Conquering Cancer*. New York: St. Martin's Press, 1981.

Welch, Deborah, and Keith Lewis. "Alopecia and Chemotherapy." *American Journal of Nursing* 80 (5) (May 1980): 903–5.

Wollard, Joy J. *Nutritional Management of the Cancer Patient*. New York: Raven Press, 1979.

MEDICAL TEXTS

Calman, Kenneth, and John Paul. *An Introduction to Cancer Medicine*. New York: John Wiley & Sons, 1978.

DeVita, Vincent, Jr., Samuel Hellman, and Steven A. Rosenberg. *Cancer: Principles and Practice of Oncology*. Philadelphia: J. B. Lippincott Co., 1982.

Frie, Emil III, and James Holland, eds. *Cancer Medicine*. Philadelphia: Lea & Febiger, 1982.

Greenspan, Ezra M., ed. *Clinical Interpretation and Practice of Cancer Chemotherapy*. New York: Raven Press, 1982.

Up-to-date information about specific forms of cancer and treatments may be found in the journals geared toward health professionals and indexed in the *Index Medicus*. This index and a selection of professional publications may be found in large public libraries and in medical libraries. Some MEDLARS centers, available at medical libraries and hospitals, will provide computer database searches for nonprofessionals. If you have trouble getting access to any of these sources, ask a physician or other health professional to help, or contact the National Cancer Institute.

BOOKLETS

The National Cancer Institute, the American Cancer Society, and many cancer centers upon request provide booklets on chemotherapy and its side effects. Especially recommended are: *Chemotherapy and You*, *Eating Hints— Recipes and Tips for Better Nutrition During Cancer Treatment*, and *Taking Time: Support for People with Cancer and People who Care about Them*.

Index

A

317

Index

Nancy Bruning has counseled cancer patients informally and was a volunteer at the Memorial Sloan-Kettering Cancer Center in New York. A writer with a particular interest in health and medicine, her previous books include SWIMMING FOR TOTAL FITNESS (with Dr. Jane Katz) and THE CONSUMER'S GUIDE TO CONTACT LENSES (with Dr. Spencer Sherman). She lives in New York.